1-21-97

Racism
Heal
Post-In

D0143624

RACISM, HEALTH, AND POST-INDUSTRIALISM

A Theory of African-American Health

Clovis E. Semmes

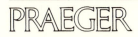

Westport, Connecticut
London

Library of Congress Cataloging-in-Publication Data

Semmes, Clovis E.
   Racism, health, and post-industrialism : a theory of African-
American health / Clovis E. Semmes.
       p. cm.
   Includes bibliographical references and index.
       ISBN 0–275–94945–1 (alk. paper).—ISBN 0–275–95428–5 (pb : alk.
paper)
       1. Afro-Americans—Health and hygiene.   2. Discrimination in
medical care—United States.   3. Afro-Americans—Social conditions.
4. Afro-Americans—Medical care.   5. Afro-Americans—Medicine.
I. Title.
RA448.5.N4S45   1996
362.1'089'96073—dc20   95–34440

British Library Cataloguing in Publication Data is available.

Library of Congress Catalog Card Number: 95–34440
ISBN: 0–275–94945–1
       0–275–95428–5 (pb.)

First published in 1996

Praeger Publishers, 88 Post Road West, Westport, CT 06881
An imprint of Greenwood Publishing Group, Inc.

Printed in the United States of America

⨂™

The paper used in this book complies with the
Permanent Paper Standard issued by the National
Information Standards Organization (Z39.48–1984).

10   9   8   7   6   5   4   3   2   1

This book is dedicated to my maternal grandmother, Raleigh Clara Smith Sales (Granny); my great-aunt, Maggie Lena Smith (Sister); and my mother, Margaret Glen Sales Semmes. Collectively, their lives affirm the healing power of love and the spirit within. For these women of wisdom, God is the ultimate healer.

Contents

Acknowledgments

Special thanks are due to Barbara Logan and Christopher Reed for their critical review of the manuscript. Charles Stevens, Bette Thompson, James Robinson, Lynn Flint, and Eastern Michigan University all provided important support for this project.

I am grateful to my wife, Jean, who read and edited numerous versions of the manuscript and who used her professional skills as a librarian to aid in the research for this work.

Thanks go to Annie Ellington, Shirley Moore, Emma Miller (Alia Al-Taqi), Cheryl Walker Cecil, and Ida Brown, who helped to gather data for various aspects of this endeavor.

Others who contributed to this book are too numerous to mention, but they have my sincere thanks and appreciation.

My children, Jelani, Maia, and Sala, continually inspire my efforts.

Introduction

This book is about how organized forms of inequality have altered, and continue to alter, the health of African Americans. It extends an earlier analysis that reveals cultural hegemony, the systemic negation of one culture by another, as a critical metaproblem challenging African-American ideational and organizational development.[1] Similarly, unusually poor trends in the health of African Americans are connected to this metaproblem. Historical, sociological, and ecological analyses reveal that the health of a people is broadly determined by the strength, resilience, and vitality of their culture.[2] As a consequence, the destructive effects of oppression and exploitation on health linger and are difficult to transcend when systemic attacks on the institutional stability of a people persist. In short, normative cultural destabilization produces added and abnormal challenges to the health status of African Americans.

To transcend this habitual and customary assault, the pursuit of health becomes both a goal and a tool of liberation. It becomes a goal because achieving better health is synonymous with transforming one's inferior status in the society. Better health is also a tool for liberation because it increases the vigor and robustness of the people. It builds and releases mental, physical, and spiritual energy that can be directed toward achieving empowerment and development. The process of self-consciously pursuing better health also attacks the fundamental mechanisms of cultural exploitation and oppression by serving to dismantle colonial-like relationships of dependency. In other words, subordinated people who actively develop and pursue an emancipatory health ethic become alert to how they are conditioned to participate in their own oppression. Thus, health consciousness becomes political consciousness.

The view that cultural viability, resilience, and effectiveness are at the center of health simultaneously complements and contrasts with the sentiment that achieving a more favorable health status for African Americans is principally a problem of gaining access to more, better, and less costly medical care. Certainly, this sentiment has validity. Moreover, the numbers of African-American medical personnel are much too low to provide an adequate foundation of medical services.[3] However, an abundance of evidence reveals that providing increasing amounts of medical care is not the most important requirement for optimum health.[4] Medicine's role, albeit an important one, has certain limits. In fact, such devastating contemporary health problems as cancer, heart disease, stroke, infant mortality, hypertension, diabetes, AIDS, and the like have a fundamental relationship to cultural fortitude and social conditions. There is a larger and more rudimentary sociocultural basis of health. Furthermore, in some instances and under certain conditions, medical care can impede the goal of health and thus requires significant restraint and reform.

Emancipatory and redemptive ideologies that have emerged from within the African-American community have frequently recognized the more essential sociocultural basis of health and the need to alter relevant cultural and institutional patterns. The National Negro Health Week initiated by Booker T. Washington and the naturalistic and alternative health care initiatives that became associated with the Black Consciousness movement of the late 1960s and 1970s are examples.[5] These movements and tendencies emerged in response to the inequality that was interwoven into the fabric of American culture, which affects health. Community-based health beliefs and practices typically embody important responses to the malaise that emanates from the experiences of human oppression, exploitation, and inequality. These experiences cannot be explained adequately by simple notions of prejudice and discrimination or as problems of cost-related access to better medical care.[6]

The goal of improving health, which involves defining sickness; establishing control over one's body; defining appropriate therapeutic procedures; specifying the parameters of mental, physical, and spiritual well-being; and the like; is continually disrupted for African Americans. The fact of historic and repeated institutional and cultural disruptions from systemic inequality challenges the normative pursuit of health. This is why the struggle for freedom and equality by African Americans is, at the same time, the struggle for health. This reality is sometimes submerged, but it is no less significant. Thus, the problem of poor health for African Americans is contextualized within the broader problem of cultural oppression. The roots of this oppression are in the evolution of the various modes of social control used in the subjugation of African peoples. The control of African labor was made possible through the use of superior weaponry and unrestrained violence, but it was perfected through the control of culture, that is, the transformation of the organizational and ideational basis of African life in the Americas.

Cultural oppression involves the concomitant misuse and misappropriation of such important institutional domains as family life, including sex and reproduction; religious thinking; identity; the organization of work; consumption; and environmental and living conditions. Each of these factors has a profound relationship to health. The shaping, reshaping, and interaction of these factors create unique, health-related accommodations for African Americans. These accommodations are further configured by the way in which structured inequality intersects the exigencies of a changing, maturing, and cyclically faltering capitalist economic order. Black labor, Black culture (particularly as it relates to consumption), White supremacy, and the context of the changing needs of Western capitalism are significant here.

The rigid exploitation of, and then the declining need for, African-American labor; the concomitant dislocation from the economy as workers; the historical restrictions on African Americans as owners-producers; and the inclining and restricted role of African Americans as consumers are essential elements for understanding the African-American health equation. The societal tendency to define the collective needs of African Americans to meet the needs of White elites further subverts internal emancipatory efforts. In this case, this means the failure to implement a transformative and liberating health ethic. Additionally, maladaptive responses by African Americans to oppression and economic dislocation become prominent, and the cultural insulation required to deflect the superexploitive machinery of a post-industrial order is diminished. This superexploitive machinery is a function of the need to expand markets in an overproduced marketplace. Weakened by a structured inequality characterized by cultural negation, the African-American community is becoming disproportionately victimized, in this era, through intensifying processes of commodification. This means that African Americans, more than other communities, are left without the necessary institutional protections to filter out external forces that produce health-negating patterns of consumption.

Other factors compound the problem. Biological and historical components and cultural adaptations that affect the nutritional status of African Americans—this includes the relationship between stress, racism, and nutrition—are important. In addition, the conditions of work and production that affect the environment (including housing), labor force participation, and the violent character of subterranean economies are significant. These factors reach into family and religious life, personal health habits, interpersonal relationships, and identity formation. As a consequence, there is a need for a more self-conscious and critical reflection on the significance of what people, institutions, and communities can and must do for themselves. This does not nullify the need for greater and less costly access to better medical care. It does, however, point to the essentially important relationship between culture and health, and also to the need to effectively comprehend the effects of structured inequality on the health-related infrastructures of African-American life.

Again, the strength, resilience, and effectiveness of one's culture, which includes how people adapt to and manage their environment, as well as their access to, and utilization of, health-related resources, is fundamental. Thus, this book examines and reveals the sociocultural foundations of health in historical context and the necessary role of health transformations in achieving human freedom and dignity.

Chapter 1 examines the relationship between social emancipation and health. It develops the idea that aggressive efforts to improve the health of an oppressed community are important steps to bring about progressive social change and empowerment. I advance the argument that, for African Americans, a profoundly critical factor affecting their health status is the continuing influence of structured inequality, which is characterized by its destabilizing effects on important health-related institutions. This phenomenon is underscored by a discussion of the fact that health is primarily a function of social and environmental factors.

Chapter 2 examines the transformations in the health of African Americans brought about by the conditions of enslavement, racial oppression, and economic exploitation. It explores the role of European expansion in altering disease vectors, changing the physical and biological environment, and disrupting institutions that are central to health.

Chapter 3 scrutinizes the conditions of antebellum life that affected health. The character of work, environmental surroundings, nutritional status, and the problem of stress in the context of a brutal system of oppression emerge as important determinants of African-American health.

Chapter 4 reveals how the same forces that impaired the health of African Americans in slavery continued in new forms and contexts during the post-slavery period. At this time, economic dislocation appeared as a new challenge to African-American health.

Chapter 5 explores the folk, popular, and alternative health care practices of African Americans. These are the indigenous efforts by African Americans to achieve better health. I examine these indigenous health practices in light of the universal need for people to understand, explain, and control the conditions of life; seek a positive cultural identity; and produce a more satisfying culture.

Chapter 6 provides an in-depth look at alternative, naturalistic health care activity in the African-American community. This activity is distinguished by its critique of the limitations of orthodox medical care and its orientation toward self-help and personal involvement in health care. It also contains the seeds of a health ethic that links constructive health behavior to collective advancement for African Americans.

Chapter 7 looks at the impact of racism, as both an ideology and an institutionalized behavior, on the delivery of medical care to African Americans. I consider the implications of the combined effects of racial inequality and the post-industrial crises of medical care for African-American health. These crises are characterized by problems of iatrogenesis (disease created by medical care) and medicalization (the tendency to expand medical markets).

Chapter 8 probes vital contemporary challenges to African-American health. I specifically examine the implications of cultural maladaptation, economic dislocation, and consumer manipulation for resolving major health problems facing African Americans. I pay particular attention to the mediating roles of family, nutrition, and stress in the struggle to enhance community health.

Chapter 9 explores ways to promote and establish a health-enhancing mode of life. I also recommend policy-related and community-based strategies to reform the distribution and delivery of orthodox medical care specifically and provide quality health care generally.

NOTES

1. Clovis E. Semmes, *Cultural Hegemony and African American Development* (Westport, Conn.: Praeger, 1992).

2. See, for example, E. Franklin Frazier, *Race and Culture Contacts in the Modern World* (Boston: Beacon Press, 1957); Todd L. Savitt, *Medicine and Slavery: The Diseases and Health of Blacks in Antebellum Virginia* (Chicago: University of Illinois Press, 1978); Kenneth F. Kiple and Virginia Himmelsteib King, *Another Dimension to the Black Diaspora: Diet, Disease, and Racism* (New York: Cambridge University Press, 1981); Franz Fanon, *Black Skin, White Mask* (New York: Grove Press, 1967).

3. My statement is not intended to be a sweeping criticism of medical-centered literature on African-American health issues. This literature provides useful and important theoretical, empirical, and policy-oriented information for improving medical services. Several excellent examples are Ronald L. Braithwaite and Sandra E. Taylor, eds., *Health Issues in the Black Community* (San Francisco: Jossey-Bass, 1992); Wornie L. Reed, *The Health and Medical Care of African-Americans: Assessment of the Status of African-Americans,* vol. 5 (Boston: University of Massachusetts at Boston, William Monroe Trotter Institute, 1992); Valiere Alcena, *The Status of the Health of Blacks in the United States of America: A Prescription for Improvement* (Dubuque, Ia.: Kendall/Hunt, 1992); Mitchell F. Rice and Woodrow Jones, Jr., eds., *Health Care Issues in Black America* (Westport, Conn.: Greenwood, 1987); Jacquelyne J. Jackson, "Urban Black Americans," in Alan Harwood, ed., *Ethnicity and Medical Care* (Cambridge, Mass.: Harvard University Press, 1981), pp. 37–129; and Ivor Lensworth Livingston, ed., *Handbook of Black American Health: The Mosaic of Conditions, Issues, Policies, and Prospects* (Westport,

Conn.: Greenwood Press, 1994). My purpose is to broaden our perspective and shift to a more holistic model of health care.

4. See, for example, John Cassel, "Psychosocial Factors in the Genesis of Disease," in Robert L. Kane, ed., *The Challenge of Community Medicine* (New York: Springer, 1974), pp. 287–300; John B. McKinlay and Sonja M. McKinlay, "Medical Measures and the Decline of Mortality," in Peter Conrad and Rochelle Kern, eds., *The Sociology of Health and Illness: Critical Perspectives,* 2d ed. (New York: St. Martin's Press, 1986), pp. 10–23; and Ivan Illich, *Medical Nemesis: The Expropriation of Health* (New York: Pantheon, 1976).

5. See Roscoe C. Brown, "The National Negro Health Week Movement," *Journal of Negro Education* 6 (July 1937): 553–564; Clovis E. Semmes, "The Role of African-American Health Beliefs and Practices in Social Movements and Cultural Revitalization," *Minority Voices* 6, no. 2 (1990): 45–57.

6. See Semmes, *Cultural Hegemony and African American Development.*

Racism,
Health, and
Post-Industrialism

1

Emancipation and the Roots of Health

The emancipatory, self-help philosophy of Booker T. Washington, the prominent late nineteenth- and early twentieth-century educator, was couched in accommodationism. It was this accommodationism, this acceptance of political subordination for African Americans, that proved most controversial and distasteful for many social reformers.[1] However, Washington's critics implicitly understood the need, by any means necessary, for a displaced and subordinated race to uplift itself. Accommodationism was a pragmatic philosophy: how could African Americans elevate themselves and transform the effects of racial oppression in the light of unrestrained White violence, economic dependency, White military superiority, and a corrupt system of justice? Of course, as W.E.B. Du Bois and others—and even Washington himself—realized, this system of inequality had to be challenged then, as it must today. The essential concerns were simply those of strategy and timing.

Washington's accommodationism, however, could not obscure the fact that he must have had an inspiring faith in the potential of a race that occupied a pitiful place in the human family after surviving over 400 years of dehumanizing servitude. It was this ability to survive, and even to prosper in the face of overwhelming odds, that gave credence to Washington's hopefulness. If one looks below the surface, the strategies of self-help, industrial education, and accommodationism implied that African Americans could never really expect a White racist society to transform itself. Emancipation could take place only as a result of the victimized transcending the conditions of oppression. There is great truth here; many oppressed people have learned that to depend on the precarious benevolence of an exploiting class is a dangerous delusion. The other side of the coin, however, is that the exploiting class, by definition, holds inordinate control over the resources of life and human advancement. Initially, these resources were taken from the oppressed, and the resulting inequality placed limits on the subordinated group's potential for self-help and self-elevation.

The lesson to be learned is that the myths of supremacy that some oppressing European groups have erected to justify their exploitation of others become inconsequential once the victimized have acquired the power of self-control, self-elevation, and self-determination. Such action is akin to the admonition, "You may not like me, but you must respect me." Similarly, paternalism and liberalism that project a language and demeanor of political correctness and racial tolerance without actually dismantling the intricacies of dependency, powerlessness, and inequality are equally hollow. Self-help and education for self-help are at the root of emancipation, as Washington, Du Bois, Marcus Garvey, Elijah Muhammad, and others would attest. Accommodation, on the other hand, is provisional and eventually may become a fetter to liberation, if reified by fear, self-doubt, and custom.

Washington's emphasis on self-help was intended to rectify the wretched condition of the culture and institutional structures of oppressed Africans in America. Poverty, illiteracy, and forced ignorance exacted a terrible toll on the quality of African-American life, as did the additional effects of violence and economic exploitation. The repercussions in health terms were enormous. Thus, a critical issue became the interrelationships between oppression, culture, and health. A slave culture—a culture of dependency, inequality, and subordination—created and perpetuated conditions that were profoundly destructive to African-American health. As a consequence, the goal of improving health logically emerged as a goal of emancipation.

Washington attempted to institutionalize this goal of improving the health of African Americans through his creation of National Negro Health Week. After observing the self-help efforts of Virginia Blacks in 1913 to enact various public health measures in their communities, Washington used Tuskegee Institute, the National Negro Business League, and his considerable prominence to advocate a program that would improve the sanitary conditions and health-related practices of African Americans.[2] What is significant here is that although Washington's efforts were adopted and supported by the federal government's Public Health Service, the impetus and momentum for the movement came from within the African-American community. Using his insight into the psychology of White supremacy, Washington secured the support of a White power structure by convincing its leaders that healthy Blacks suited their economic interest.[3] Again, the pragmatic reality was that this power structure saw little reason to assist its victims unless there was some significant return on the

dollar. African Americans are all too familiar with the problem of meas-
uring their own intrinsic value and human worth based upon the needs
and greed of others.

Another problem was the continuing myth that the sordid conditions of
African Americans were somehow racially determined. Blacks, of course,
wanted to explode this myth, but a White supremacist society saw vindi-
cation in its perpetuation. One biographer of W.E.B. Du Bois illustrated
this perspective when he noted that at the conference inaugurating the
famous Atlanta sociological studies on African Americans, a White professor, Eugene Harris, from Fisk University pronounced, "The suppression of his ballot, and the other discriminations that are made against the
black man, have at least no immediate bearing on his health, vitality, or
longevity."[4] This warped declaration was challenged by Du Bois's massive
and groundbreaking work, *The Philadelphia Negro*. Du Bois later commented in one of his own biographical accounts that *The Philadelphia
Negro* "revealed the Negro group as a symptom, not a cause; as a striving,
palpitating group, and not an inert, sick body of crime; as a losing historic
development and not a transient occurrence."[5]

Du Bois, as did other African-American scholars, understood that the
causes of Black deprivation were environmental and not racial (that is,
somehow residing in the genes). Further, if there was a failing of culture,
the cause was exploitation and oppression and not an innate inability to
construct a workable mode of life. Nevertheless, the symbolic structures
of White supremacy systemically erect and reproduce built-in exonerations
for its historic crimes and complicity in Black subordination. Washington
may have avoided criticizing the racism of White elites, but he knew, as
did Du Bois, that its victims had to be agents for change and bring about
their own liberation.

For people who must address the problem of cultural oppression, movement toward self-determination, self-help, liberation, and the like necessarily requires a critical assessment of the conditions affecting their health
and well-being. The African-American experience, of course, exemplifies
the universal truth that positive health outcomes are integrally related to
the intersection of social organization and culture. By this I mean that the
quality of health proceeds significantly from the manner in which people
are able to organize their lives in relationship to acquiring and utilizing
available and needed resources for survival and prosperity. The precise
way in which this is done—its institutionalization in the context of extant
beliefs, values, and norms—constitutes the dynamics of a culture of health.
These health-related patterns can, and should, act as guides that ensure
the relative and potential well-being of current and future generations.
The persistently poor health of African Americans relative to White
Americans is a testimony to the tenacity of perennial disruptions to African-American institutional life. It also reflects the dependency—psycho-

logical and economic—produced by centuries of exploitation and structured inequality. For African Americans, access to quality health care has been, and continues to be, affected by the pressures of institutionalized inequality, but this fact must be understood in the context of the social basis of health and the limitations of medical care.

THE SOCIAL BASIS OF HEALTH

As societies have shifted from agricultural to industrial (and post-industrial) forms, the struggle against disease has shifted from a principal concern with infectious and parasitic diseases to a greater concern with chronic and degenerative ailments. Thus, as the ravages of malaria, yellow fever, tuberculosis, syphilis, parasitic worms, diphtheria, and similar diseases have declined, the problems of cancer, heart disease, diabetes, hypertension, and the like have increased. Modern or scientific medicine developed effective methods of treatment against invading microorganisms, parasites, and disease-carrying insects and animals through antibiotics, immunizations, and other powerful drugs. Furthermore, it made significant strides in diagnosis, the control of pain, and corrective and reconstructive surgery. In consequence, our faith in medicine to fix health problems grew and the misconception that health is primarily a function of medical care was enhanced.[6]

With the emergence of a germ theory of disease, which identified discrete and independent disease-causing organisms that could be eradicated, the dominant cultural view became the belief that modern medicine literally could attack disease.[7] This model of disease causation heightened the validation of a biomedical treatment model, which applied an engineering approach to curing sick bodies. Using this model, physicians saw the body as a machine that could be manipulated through both chemical and surgical intervention and radiation. Additionally, the tendency to separate psychological processes from biological ones—a philosophical stance that had already become a cornerstone of Western positivist science—further contributed to an epistemological reduction of the body to a machine-like object that could be managed, thus severing its ecological and metaphysical connections. One consequence was to ignore the importance of the body's ability to resist infection and the myriad of social factors that contribute to resistance against disease.

The importance of social factors in disease resistance and health promotion is reflected in the fact that despite modern medicine's diagnostic and curative competence, it did not initiate the downward trends in infectious and parasitic diseases or stimulate the dramatic increases in human longevity. Diseases like polio, diphtheria, and tuberculosis were beginning to show significant declines prior to the development and utilization of effective treatments by modern medicine. Similarly, cholera, typhoid, and dysentery reached their peak and began to decline independent of medical control. In the second half of the nineteenth century, U.S. deaths from childhood diseases began to decline before the introduction of antibiotics and widespread immunization.[8] Increased human longevity was linked to dramatic declines in infant mortality, and clearly, the progress of modern medicine was not responsible for the decline in mortality from the 1900s onward.[9] Indeed, we find that "with a few exceptions, the technical advances of modern medicine have not led to major improvements in measures of health, illness, life expectancy, or death."[10] The key components in the achievement of better health have been improved sanitation and nutrition and the resulting stabilization of births. Environmental adaptation, in its broadest sense, is the principal determinant of the health of any population.[11]

Psychosocial Factors and Health

The importance of the body's resistance in mitigating disease and in health promotion also directs greater attention to the role of psychosocial factors. For example, population changes that destabilize social settings, group membership, and the quality of group relations can produce changes in the neuroendocrine system which, in turn, heighten susceptibility to disease.[12] Such heightened physiological disequilibriums are found in the disruptive effects of urban migration and industrialization on rural populations and the disruptive effects of post-urban downsizing and economic dislocation on established urban populations. Subordinate groups experience the most extreme health-threatening reactions to severe social change, but social supports, such as fully functioning families, provide a great measure of protection against disease-enhancing flux.[13]

Infectious and parasitic diseases and chronic and degenerative ailments are typically influenced by shifting social and environmental conditions and the institutional capability to respond suitably to those conditions. Medical care is one element of that response, but it is not a decisive determinant of health. Primary prevention, when possible, is superior to secondary and tertiary prevention. Primary prevention means taking steps to prevent disease. Secondary prevention involves early action to minimize the seriousness of the disease process. It includes screening and early detection. Tertiary prevention is the effort, through clinical medicine, to minimize the complications of an established disease process.[14] Primary prevention is the most cost-effective health promotion strategy and is strongly connected to cultural traditions. An appropriate proactive social response can lead to the reduced virulence and incidence of infectious diseases and to the prevention, effective management, or reversal of degenerative and chronic ailments. Degenerative and chronic health problems are, for example, sensitive to lifestyle, a process that is embedded in family functioning and other forms of institutional behavior. In addition, there are broader environmental issues that involve the effective management of toxic waste and the rapid erosion of life-giving and health-enhancing ecological systems.

Environmental Toxicity and Health

Industrialization, modernization, and the internal dynamics of a post-industrial economic system that superexploits natural resources and markets exacerbate problems of ecological damage and toxic waste production. Tropical rain forests, which are estimated to contain 50 percent of the world's biological species, are being cut down at the rate of one acre per second.[15] Because of expanding industrial production, millions of people breath dangerously high levels of ozone, which damages the respiratory passages. Ozone-destroying chlorofluorocarbons released into the stratosphere diminish protection from the sun's harmful ultraviolet rays.[16] Sulfur dioxide from the combustion of fossil fuels like coal and crude oil contributes to bronchial constriction and lung disease. In addition, particulate air pollution (the particles remaining suspended in the air after any form of combustion) is associated with increased mortality.[17]

The environmental health hazards produced by industrial production disproportionately affect African Americans. Blacks are overrepresented in "high-risk" occupations, which frequently expose them to toxic chemicals, and African-American communities are more likely than other communities to be located near dumping grounds for municipal refuse and toxic waste. A history of racial oppression has relegated African Americans to greater economic dependency and political powerlessness which, in turn, increase the probability that they will live and work under conditions plagued by higher levels of disease-causing toxicity.[18]

On April 15, 1987, a landmark study on demographic patterns associated with hazardous waste sites was released by the United Church of Christ Commission for Racial Justice at the National Press Club in Washington, D.C. Dr. Benjamin Chavis, Jr., was the executive director of the commission at the time. As a consequence of the study's findings, he coined the term "environmental racism."[19] Leading scholars on environmental racism have concluded that there is "clear and unequivocal evidence that income and racial biases in the distribution of environmental hazards exist" and that "race is more importantly related to the distribution of these hazards than income."[20]

Lifestyle and Health

The social basis of health is further revealed through a growing awareness of the relationship between lifestyle and health.[21] For example, there are strong correlations between what we consume and do to our bodies and significant increases in degenerative and chronic diseases. The solid and consistent correlations between, on the one hand, smoking cigarettes or consuming diets high in fat with, on the other, increased rates of cancer are examples.[22] Alcohol consumption contributes to a wide range of chronic and degenerative health problems. It also is associated with nearly half of all homicides and with a large proportion of accidental injuries. Cancer of the esophagus and cirrhosis of the liver are other effects of alcohol use.[23] Research has shown that in some cases, obesity and super-obesity are strongly associated with sedentary lifestyles characterized by excessive television viewing.[24] For African Americans, for example, life-style and dietary factors play a significant role in persistently high rates of hypertension.[25]

A limitation of the lifestyle focus, however, is the emphasis on changing discrete personal behaviors. Even though such conduct as smoking, eating the wrong foods, engaging in high-risk behaviors (for example, unpro-tected sex), and the failure to use safety devices like seat belts is individ-ualistic, such behavior must be understood in much broader interactional circumstances. Cocaine use, for example, is embedded within a multiplicity of interrelated, unhealthy habits and behaviors. Cocaine users have poorer diets, tend to consume more alcohol, and engage in fewer stress-reducing activities than nonusers.[26] People in poverty who suddenly are able to spend more on food may not eat more nutritiously because of strongly embedded cultural habits. Moreover, eating has other social functions be-sides nutrition. It may be connected to religious doctrine, aesthetic norms, or social status.[27] Focusing only on the distinct behaviors of individuals obscures societal factors that are more crucial to effective health promo-tion. Thus, personal health behavior must be understood in its sociocul-tural and institutional contexts.[28]

Family and Health

One of the most important institutional contexts in which to understand the lifestyle determinants of disease is the family. It is usually in the family that at-risk behavior is learned, supported, or reduced. In addition, the family provides the principal coping mechanism for mediating, mitigating, and diffusing stress. Sustained stress can contribute significantly to poor health and illness by weakening the immune response, heightening nutri-tional needs, or stimulating extant disease processes.[29] Family members influence each other's health through developing and sharing similar pat-terns of eating, and they tend to engage in kindred at-risk behaviors. For example, the consumption of sodium-rich diets and obesity, which are both important risk factors in contracting hypertension, are found to be more prevalent in pre-teenage African-American girls who have obese mothers who consume sodium-rich diets.[30] Smokers tend to marry smokers, and obese people tend to marry obese people. Family members tend also to develop similar orientations toward physical fitness, and parental patterns of health care use are a good predictor of the children's use of health care.[31]

It is likely that at-risk behaviors are much more difficult to change if they are shared by others in the family.[32] This is because health-related behaviors have strongly rooted social functions. For example, patterns of food preparation and eating may be used to reward, show love to, or control others. What a family eats affirms common values and helps to define the identity of the group. Eating, smoking, and the use of alcohol have a role in patterns of sociability and methods of coping with stress. Thus, when one person attempts to alter his or her lifestyle, there is a rippling effect on others in the family. As a consequence, there may be both overt and covert resistance and resentment. In a addition, if lifestyle change is to take place, there must be a model for change. If such a model is lacking in the family, individual change becomes much more difficult. In short, health promotion becomes a problem of how to deconstruct an old way of life and construct a new one.[33]

The family can either promote or impede health, but it usually does both under varying conditions and situations. Families handle most health problems. Without this function, formal health care systems would be hopelessly overburdened.[34] Thus, the quality of care given and the health care decisions made within the family are extremely important. For example, the involvement of a spouse can enhance how the other spouse may control hypertension. However, the more decisive set of family behaviors are those related to preventive and health-enhancing activity, of which dietary habits, the removal or minimalization of at-risk behaviors, and the development and maintenance of effective coping mechanisms are examples.

The importance of the viability of the family to the health of its members suggests a special burden on single-parent families. For example, research indicates that single motherhood is a significant risk factor when it comes to the health of the children. The higher rates of poverty and the absence of adequate social supports for single mothers are the important factors that mitigate the health-enhancing vitality of this family type.[35]

Through their ability to provide social support, families can improve their members' health. For example, marriage has a protective effect; it reduces the incidence and virulence of disease and increases longevity. Moreover, the presence of children tends to help the elderly live longer. Another example of the supportive potential of the family is how it addresses the experience of losing a loved one (bereavement). Bereavement, through its relationship to stress and at-risk coping behavior (smoking, alcohol and drug use, and eating and sleeping patterns), can lead to illness.[36] A family that consciously promotes a culture of health is better able to develop a progressive and proactive route to managing stress-producing and disease-enhancing crises. One way in which health consciousness is cultivated and sustained in the family is through religious and sacred beliefs.

Religion and Health

Religious and sacred beliefs have a profound effect on the complexity of factors that constitute the social basis of health. Sacred beliefs are special beliefs because of their relative strength and importance in shaping human behavior. They are usually tied to some religious system, whether formal or informal; alternately, they are simply maintained as fundamental understandings about social and cosmological order, cause and effect, life and death, and similar phenomena. Religious participation brings with it forms of sociability that reinforce diverse types of health behavior. For example, social gatherings imply normative acceptance and expectations regarding categories and quantities of food consumption. Sacred and religious beliefs also embody conceptual and explanatory models regarding the causes and sources of disease and poor health. What people believe to be the cause of disease and poor health will determine to a large degree the particular solutions they will seek.[37]

Historically and cross-culturally, religious and sacred beliefs and health beliefs and practices have always been connected because of the fundamental belief that life, healing, and death are ultimately related to a higher creative force or being. Groups use religious beliefs to explain the causes of disease and to seek cures, usually through divine intervention but also through the use of herbal remedies, dietary practices, and other therapeutic modalities associated with these beliefs. In a broad spectrum of cultures, religious and spiritual leaders are also expected to be adept as healers. In other cultural contexts, the role of healer is only marginally claimed by religious and spiritual principals. We must recognize that religious and sacred explanatory models of health and illness are central to the well-being of groups, not only because of how such beliefs may affect the way in which individuals seek formalized health care and interact with health professionals, but, in a more important way, in how they affect the way in which individuals perceive and encounter life itself and how they engage in self-help health practices.

One way that we can expect the cognitive dimensions of religious and sacred beliefs to affect health is through their relationship to managing stress, which plays a role in stimulating disease processes. Religious and sacred beliefs can function to mitigate stress by mediating how one perceives the exigencies of life, the inevitability of death, the meaning of existence, and the management of interpersonal relationships. Religious ritual, fellowship, or involvement in a community of believers can be an important vehicle for dispelling stress. Activities that involve prayer, meditation, singing, and dancing—individually or collectively—can be therapeutic and can heighten belief in the potential for cure. Thus, through stress reduction, religious and sacred activity can act as powerful forms of preventive health care and contribute to reducing the virulence of disease processes. Others to whom one is connected through shared sacred beliefs and rituals can become potent forms of social support. They, in effect, become an extended family, which forms a vehicle for mutual aid.[38]

Another way in which religious and sacred beliefs can have a positive effect on health is through the way they strengthen family life and contribute to the transmission of important health-related values and behaviors. Strongly held religious and sacred beliefs, for example, can help sustain family functioning in the face of disintegrating social forces brought about by poverty and economic dislocation. Sacred beliefs that affect dietary habits and at-risk behaviors like smoking and alcohol consumption can serve as critical preventive health measures. Through the family, varieties of behaviors are handed down—in the context of religious and sacred beliefs—that impart important health-related knowledge and practices about childbirth, child rearing, breast-feeding, sexual activity, fitness, and developing an organized and balanced mode of life.[39]

In contrast, sacred and religious beliefs also may impede the goal of health by inadequately addressing health issues or by promoting modes of life that are potentially destructive to one's health. Norms regarding dietary habits and sociability easily come to mind, but some religious beliefs and practices may direct groups away from taking responsibility for their health. The belief that everything is in God's hands may suggest to some people that they can do little to affect their health status. Certain religious and sacred doctrines also may tie individuals into belief systems that cause them to question their own human worth and value. Racism and sexism embodied in religious beliefs are examples, and the internalization of such beliefs by oppressed groups may reinforce their malleability to the health-destroying manipulations of oppressing groups.[40] It is also the case that sacred beliefs may include beliefs and practices that are intended to be health promoting, yet, because of situational and conditional factors, the opposite effect is achieved.[41]

VIEWING HEALTH HOLISTICALLY

In an effort to understand the determinants of health, the Western medical tradition has postulated a biomedical model that stresses manipulating the physiology of the body. Researchers later began to recognize the psychosocial dimensions of health, which highlight the mediating influences of social processes in determining health. For example, the relationship between stress and disease processes is prominent. The further elaboration of the psychosocial approach emphasizes the central role of the family in the health of individuals, groups, and communities. In recognition of biomedical and psychosocial determinants of health, scholars constructed the biopsychosocial model.[42] However, it does not adequately address religious, spiritual, and metaphysical realities.

Phenomena that exist outside mainstream Western scientistic empiricism are experienced by many groups.[43] As a consequence, viewing religious, spiritual, and metaphysical realities only as beliefs, as opposed to active, causative agents in health maintenance, is too reductionist. What emerges for non-Western cultures and various nonmainstream ethnic and racial groups within Western societies is a biopsychosocial-spiritual model of health care. Asian and African approaches to health care that posit the existence and importance of a life force, the importance of mind (consciousness and awareness) in directing this life force, and the need to address interconnected spiritual phenomena regarding one's relationship to God, nature, ancestors, and other spiritual agents provide a more expanded, integrated, and high-context conception of healing and curing. I do not mean that such approaches do not operate in Western cultures, but they are not central to the dominant mode of belief directing Western health promotion and care.

One may argue that such issues are subsumed under the psychosocial aspects of health care, but a biopsychosocial-spiritual model represents a shift away from a linear perspective that is discrete and additive. This model represents a shift to an integrated and holistic approach that is indivisible in terms of the issues one must address to sustain health. In fact, the causal emphasis within such a model moves back and forth and occurs reflexively. Health-sustaining activity and the healing and curative approaches that tend to balance the biochemistry of the body, thus strengthening and balancing the body's life force, affecting the way in which people think, harmonizing interpersonal relationships, reintegrating people into family and community life, and promoting health arts are examples of such holism. The recognition of the functional importance of a biopsychosocial-spiritual role in human existence should also help to revitalize the health of African Americans because it calls for greater integration and self-conscious reflection of African-American cultural needs and realities.

If we understand broad social processes affecting health, which include how groups address religious, spiritual, and metaphysical realities, the character of community life emerges as an added determinant. Community life nourishes and supports the culture of groups and has the capacity to sustain, enhance, or impede the health-promoting activities of everyday life. It is through the community that a health ethic is disseminated and preserved. By health ethic I mean traditions that contribute to the institutional strength of a community such that they can provide insulation against external, health-negating forces and internally generate a pervasively health-enhancing mode of life. As a consequence, the community will become empowered and can resist exploitive forces. The need for specialized health practitioners and services is not negated, but the burden of health maintenance is shifted to where it is most efficient and effective, within the context of the institutional life of the community. This shift in emphasis should also increase the accountability and responsiveness of health providers, hold down health care costs, and increase positive indicators of health.

CULTURAL HEGEMONY AND HEALTH

A crucial problem for African Americans is the unique way in which they have become connected to the American social order. After they were kidnapped from Africa and exploited as a cheap source of labor, their European oppressors found that the systematic disruption and destabilization of African cultures was the most efficient and effective way to control the captive population. We can contrast this mode of oppression with the genocidal acts committed against Native peoples and their subsequent confinement to reservations. Both groups were assaulted culturally, but the goals were to deprive Native peoples of their land and Africans of their labor.

When the economic needs of European American enclaves of power changed to the point where the enslavement of Africans was no longer needed, the question of what to do with peoples of African descent became a central issue in shaping the entire fabric of American life and culture. The Civil Rights movements of the 1950s and 1960s were an expression of this controversy as African Americans challenged a White settler colony that never intended to include non-White peoples in its social order. Additionally, the culture of African Americans is expropriated by White enclaves of power to fuel the popular culture that is essential to drive America's market system domestically and globally—a process that is becoming increasingly more exploitive and essential in response to intensifying post-industrial constraints to economic growth. The same processes of cultural negation that were useful to create a supply of compliant slave labor functioned to perpetuate maladaptation and institutional and cultural weaknesses among African Americans. Cultural hegemony emerged as a metaproblem, and in this post-industrial era, the perpetuation of cultural dependency heightens the potential for market penetration and radical consumer exploitation.

What, then, are the health implications of this dynamic? Quite simply, African-American communities are faced with systemic, day-to-day realities that tend to reward them for serving the economic, political, and cultural interests of White enclaves of power. These realities tend to punish and delegitimate self-conscious actions designed to elevate and empower African Americans as a group. As a consequence, if we understand that health is much more sensitive and responsive to cultural configurations than it is to systems of sick care, the implications of the problem of cultural hegemony should become clear. Cultural dependency leaves the African-American community much less protected than other groups and, therefore, overly exposed to greater amounts of health-negating consumer manipulation and exploitation.

"Cultural hegemony, the fundamental vehicle of systemic White supremacy, tends to deprive African Americans of a sustained capacity to develop a social and spiritual ethic that can serve their collective needs."[44] This does not mean, however, that there are not times when the goals and objectives of White enclaves of power correspond to certain collective goals and needs of African Americans. Also, White enclaves of power are not monolithic and do compete with one another for political, economic, and cultural ascendancy. However, if the problem of African-American cultural dependency resulting from the metaproblem of cultural hegemony is not addressed, what will happen when the health needs of an African-American collective run counter to the economic and cultural priorities of powerful White elites?

An African-American–centered health perspective is needed to drive a functional and progressive health ethic. Such a perspective must draw on a historical and deep cultural analysis of African Americans and their relationship to the American social order. The result should be to provide a progressive, interpretive framework for discerning actions and policies that function to serve the comprehensive health needs of African Americans. Such a framework should also enhance our understanding of how to improve the health of all Americans. However, for African Americans, because of their unique history and connections to American society, there must be the added step of dismantling destructive and destabilizing societal relationships that impede and distort their efforts to produce a more functional and progressive culture. This culture must serve to elevate the health status of African Americans.

NOTES

1. See, for example, the discussion of Booker T. Washington in W.E.B. Du Bois, *The Souls of Black Folk* (Greenwich, Conn.: Fawcett, 1961), pp. 42–54.

2. See James H. Jones, *Bad Blood: The Tuskegee Syphilis Experiment—A Tragedy of Race and Medicine* (New York: Free Press, 1981), pp. 34–35.

3. See Roscoe C. Brown, "The National Negro Health Week Movement," *Journal of Negro Education* 6 (July 1937): 553–564.

4. A former student, Annie Ellington, pointed out this statement in David

Lewis Levering, *W.E.B. Du Bois: Biography of a Race 1868–1919* (New York: Henry Holt, 1993), p. 219.

5. W.E.B. Du Bois, *Dusk of Dawn: An Essay toward an Autobiography of a Race Concept* (New York: Schocken, 1968), p. 59.

6. See John Powles, "On the Limitations of Modern Medicine," in Robert L. Kane, ed., *The Challenge of Community Medicine* (New York: Springer, 1974), pp. 89–122; and Ivan Illich, *Medical Nemesis: The Expropriation of Health* (New York: Pantheon, 1976).

7. Powles, "On the Limitations of Modern Medicine," pp. 103–106.

8. Illich, *Medical Nemesis,* pp. 13–16; John Cassel, "Psychological Factors in the Genesis of Disease," in Robert L. Kane, ed., *The Challenge of Community Medicine* (New York: Springer, 1974), p. 287.

9. John B. McKinlay and Sonja M. McKinlay, "Medical Measures and the Decline of Mortality," in Peter Conrad and Rochelle Kern, eds., *The Sociology of Health and Illness: Critical Perspectives,* 2d ed. (New York: St. Martin's Press, 1986), pp. 10–23.

10. Howard Waitzkin, *The Second Sickness: Contradictions of Capitalist Health Care* (New York: Free Press, 1983), p. 28.

11. Illich, *Medical Nemesis,* p. 17; Waitzkin, *The Second Sickness,* p. 28; Powles, "On the Limitations of Modern Medicine," p. 96.

12. Cassel, "Psychosocial Factors in the Genesis of Disease," p. 296.

13. Ibid., pp. 290–294; Leonard A. Sagan, *The Health of Nations: True Causes of Sickness and Well-Being* (New York: Basic Books, 1987), pp. 110, 128.

14. Robert L. Kane, "Disease Control: What Is Really Preventable?" in Robert L. Kane, ed., *The Challenge of Community Medicine* (New York: Springer, 1974), pp. 123–124.

15. Anthony D. Cortese, "Introduction: Human Health, Risk, and the Environment," in Eric Chivian, Michael McCally, Howard Hu, and Andrew Haines, eds., *Critical Condition: Human Health and the Environment* (Cambridge, Mass.: Massachusetts Institute of Technology Press, 1993), p. 3.

16. Ibid., pp. 2–3.

17. David C. Christiani, "Urban and Transboundary Air Pollution: Human Health Consequences," in Eric Chivian, Michael McCally, Howard Hu, and Andrew Haines, eds., *Critical Condition: Human Health and the Environment* (Cambridge, Mass.: Massachusetts Institute of Technology Press, 1993), pp. 16–18.

18. James H. Johnson, Jr., and Melvin L. Oliver, "Blacks and the Toxic Crisis," *Western Journal of Black Studies* 13, no. 2 (1989): 72–78; Beverly Hendrix Wright and Robert Bullard, "Hazards in the Workplace and Black Health," *National Journal of Sociology* 4 (Spring 1990): 45–62.

19. Charles Lee, "Toxic Waste and Race in the United States," in Bunyan Bryant and Paul Mohai, eds., *Race and the Incidence of Environmental Hazards: A Time for Discourse* (Boulder, Colo.: Westview Press, 1992), p. 10.

20. Paul Mohai and Bunyan Bryant, "Environmental Racism: Reviewing the Evidence," in Bunyan Bryant and Paul Mohai, eds., *Race and the Incidence of Environmental Hazards: A Time for Discourse* (Boulder, Colo.: Westview Press, 1992), p. 174.

21. World Health Organization, Health Education Unit, Regional Office for

Europe, "Life-Styles and Health," *Social Science and Medicine* 22, no. 2 (1986): 117–124.

22. George Berkley, *On Being Black and Healthy: How Black Americans Can Lead Longer and Healthier Lives* (Englewood Cliffs, N.J.: Prentice-Hall, 1982), p. 50; Claudia R. Baquet and Tyson Gibbs, "Cancer and Black Americans," in Ronald L. Braithwaite and Sandra E. Taylor, eds., *Health Issues in the Black Community* (San Francisco: Jossey-Bass, 1992), pp. 109–110.

23. National Research Council Committee on the Status of Black Americans, *A Common Destiny: Blacks and American Society* (Washington, D.C.: National Academy Press, 1989), pp. 414–415.

24. Larry A. Tucker and Glenn M. Friedman, "Television Viewing and Obesity in Adult Males," *American Journal of Public Health* 79 (April 1989): 516–518.

25. Ivor L. Livingston, "Blacks, Life-Style and Hypertension: The Importance of Health Education," *Humboldt Journal of Social Relations* 14 (Fall/Winter 1986; Spring/Summer 1987): 195–213.

26. Felipe G. Castro, Michael D. Newcomb, and Karen Cadish, "Lifestyle Differences between Young Adult Cocaine Users and Nonuser Peers," *Journal of Drug Education* 17, no. 2 (1987): 89–111.

27. Alan Berg, *The Nutrition Factor: Its Role in National Development* (Washington, D.C.: Brookings Institution, 1973), p. 44.

28. Jeannine Coreil, Jeffrey S. Levin, and E. Gartly Jaco, "Life Style—An Emergent Concept in the Sociomedical Sciences," *Culture, Medicine and Psychiatry* 9, no. 4 (1985): 423–437.

29. William J. Doherty and Thomas L. Campbell, *Families and Health* (Beverly Hills, Calif.: Sage, 1988), pp. 22–25.

30. Robert J. Karp, Clara Williams, and Jeanne-Olivia Grant, "Increased Utilization of Salty Food with Age among Preteenage Black Girls," *Journal of the National Medical Association* 72, no. 3 (1980): 197–200.

31. Doherty and Campbell, *Families and Health*, pp. 32–33.

32. Ibid.

33. Ibid., pp. 34–35; see also, for example, Clovis E. Semmes, "When Medicine Fails: Making the Decision to Seek Natural Health Care," *National Journal of Sociology* 4, no. 2 (Fall 1990): 175–198.

34. Doherty and Campbell, *Families and Health*, p. 69.

35. Ronald Angel and Jacqueline Lowe Worobey, "Single Motherhood and Children's Health," *Journal of Health and Social Behavior* 29 (March 1988): 38–52.

36. Ibid., pp. 52–56.

37. See for example, Edward H. Spicer, ed., *Ethnic Medicine in the Southwest* (Tucson: University of Arizona Press, 1977).

38. See, for example, Clovis E. Semmes "Toward a Theory of Popular Health Practices in the Black Community," *Western Journal of Black Studies* 7, no. 4 (1983): 206–213; Migene González-Wippler, *Santeria: African Magic in Latin America* (New York: Original Publications, 1987); Meredith B. McGuire, *Ritual Healing in Suburban America* (New Brunswick, N.J.: Rutgers University Press, 1988); and Fred M. Frohock, *Healing Powers: Alternative Medicine, Spiritual Communities and the State* (Chicago: University of Chicago Press, 1992).

39. See Henry Troyer, "Review of Cancer among 4 Religious Sects: Evidence

That Life-styles Are Distinctive Sets of Risk Factors," *Social Science and Medicine* 26, no. 10 (1988): 1007–1017; and Clovis E. Semmes, "The Role of African-American Health Beliefs and Practices in Social Movements and Cultural Revitalization," *Minority Voices* 6, no. 2 (Spring 1990): 45–57.

40. See Clovis E. Semmes, *Cultural Hegemony and African American Development* (Westport, Conn.: Praeger, 1992), pp. 138–169.

41. See, for example, Steven Bachrach, Julian Fisher, and John S. Parks, "An Outbreak of Vitamin D Deficiency Rickets in a Susceptible Population," *Pediatrics* 64, no. 6 (December 1979): 871–877.

42. Doherty and Campbell, *Families and Health,* p. 14.

43. See, for example, Spicer, *Ethnic Medicine in the Southwest;* Arthur Kleinman, *Patients and Healers in the Context of Culture* (Los Angeles: University of California Press, 1980).

44. Semmes, *Cultural Hegemony,* p. 172.

2

Race and Culture Contact and the
Equilibrium of Health

E. Franklin Frazier's classic study, *Race and Culture Contact in the Modern World,* examines the ecology of racial oppression and in doing so provides important insights into the social and cultural basis of health. He noted that the ecological basis of race relations involves the manner in which one group relates to its environment affects other groups with different racial and cultural backgrounds.[1] Specifically, Frazier argued that European expansion and its associated methods of environmental exploitation adversely affected non-European peoples. Europeans altered how non-European groups related to their environments and transformed the internal social relations of these groups. The results were a myriad of health problems. For Africans in the Americas and for Native Americans and others, these health problems presented tremendous obstacles to survival and group development. Moreover, in many instances, these obstacles formed the foundation for contemporary health crises.

The European search for wealth that precipitated contact with Africa in the fifteenth century would forever tie the African Americans' intragroup social and ecological relations to the changing exigencies of European American ecological adaptations and modes of achieving economic goals. A simple, but by no means isolated, example is chattel slavery.[2] A subsequent and continually evolving issue is the decline in the need for African-American labor.[3]

NEW WORLD CONTACT

Frazier noted that Marco Polo's accounts of his travels in eastern Asia during the thirteenth century awakened the imagination of the European populace and broadened its view of the world.[4] This imagination became dominated by the desire for new riches and wealth, to be appropriated in the name of a European god. The proselytizing zeal and belief in the inferiority and defective condition of non-Christian cultures carried by European Christian missionaries was to become the normative context by which all Europeans would view peoples not like themselves. The missionaries became the advanced guard for economic and political domination and helped to justify violence and terror as a means of extracting the wealth, land, and labor of others.

Ultimately, European nations laid waste to the indigenous cultures of the new lands they visited and established White settler colonies in such places as North, South, and Central America; the West Indies; Australia; New Zealand; and South Africa. The devastating turning point for Africa's humanity was the exploration and subjugation of key African coastal regions by the Portuguese in the early fifteenth century and the Spanish-backed voyages of Columbus to the New World in 1492. The intersection of religious intolerance and greed produced full-blown ideologies of European or White supremacy.[5]

As Europe looked for effective ways to extract the wealth of new lands, it consciously and unconsciously transmuted the life chances and social and ecological relations of non-European peoples in general and Africans in particular. The introduction or spread of various new and extant plant and animal life; the introduction of firearms, strong alcoholic drinks, and new microbes; the transformation and destruction of traditional forms of social organization; the disruption of nutritional environments; the stimulation of significant population upheavals; the implementation of a culture of cruelty and violence; and the emergence of a psychology of oppression are some of the effects of changes in the European ecological relationships.

THE EVOLUTION OF AFRICAN ENSLAVEMENT

Sugar production and the evolution of massive African enslavement provide some illustration of how human relations and health were refashioned by new ecological adaptations and challenges. As a consequence of the Crusades—the extended struggle between European Christendom and Muslims for the control of Palestine—Europeans had established sugar plantations using slave labor in parts of Syria and Palestine.[6] As we are informed by Drake, slavery was not confined to a particular racial group, and the Christians frequently used, among others, Syrian and Arab prisoners of war.[7] Eastern Europeans were also objects of the brisk sale of humans around the Mediterranean and, in fact, from their name, *Slavs,* the designation *slave* was born.[8] However, as Muslim strength became too great, Europeans shifted their sugar plantations westward to Crete, Cyprus, and Sicily.[9] Cyprus became the largest slave market in the Mediter-ranean, with slaves including Greeks, Jews and other Whites, and a few Blacks.[10] Invading Turks eventually forced the movement of European sugar production to Spain and then Portugal, and finally to islands off the coast of Africa. In this new environment, the number of African slaves increased, but multiracial slavery was still the norm. Drake explained:

The decisive event increasing the flow of sub-Saharan Blacks into the Mediterra-nean labor pool was the victory of the Ottoman Turks over the Byzantine Christian empire which included the seizure of Constantinople in 1453. With the flow of White slaves from Russian diminishing, the demand for sub-Saharan Blacks, as well as prisoners of war from all ethnic groups, increased sharply. . . . [I]nvestors moved the industry to the offshore islands of Madeira, the Canarie, Cape Verde, and then Fernando Po and São Tome off the coast of Nigeria.[11]

The next phase of this historical process would be the transfer of sugar production to the Caribbean in the early sixteenth century, but this did not occur until after the Portuguese had established a monopoly on the human trade in Africans, beginning in the fifteenth century. The stage was set for establishing this monopoly when the Portuguese captured the Mor-occan port of Ceuta in 1415. This was the first acquisition of African ter-ritory by the Portuguese, and it became the initial step toward Portuguese colonial expansion.[12] The capture of Ceuta was led by Prince Henry of Portugal, who was later known as Prince Henry the Navigator.[13] Subse-quently, the Portuguese continued their exploration off the coast of West Africa as they sailed southward. In 1441, the Portuguese captain, Antão Goncalvez, who was in the service of Prince Henry, seized ten Africans from Cape Borjador.[14] These Africans were presented to Prince Henry, who in turn presented them to Pope Martin V. The pope was moved to sanction the capture of Africans and to confer sovereignty upon any pos-session taken by the Portuguese in Guinea.[15] Other Africans had been seized and sold in Europe by 1444, but by 1460, 700 to 800 Africans were enslaved and carried to Portugal for sale annually.[16]

The flood gates of African slavery were not to open until the middle of the sixteenth century, however, and the resulting sea of human misery was directly related to the Columbian voyage of 1492. First, however, in the New World was the misery of the Arawak and Carib peoples. The Spanish encountered islands in the West Indies that were abundantly populated with a peaceful and healthy humanity.[17] However, almost from the very beginning, the conquerors implemented a policy of unrestrained cruelty.[18] Columbus, for example, had no problems ordering his soldiers to seize men, women, and children from their homes and, indicative of Spanish contempt for their amiable hosts, Columbus made reference in his journal to seizing "seven head of women," as if they were livestock.[19]

Armed with superior weaponry, greed, and religious justification, the Spanish subjugated the Native people and furiously searched for precious metals. This enslavement, search, and seizure process was to extend throughout the sixteenth century to other areas of the New World; the Spanish, for example, ultimately were to destroy the Aztec civilization of central Mexico and the Inca civilization of Peru, places that yielded extraordinary quantities of gold, silver, and other precious metals.[20] However, in the West Indies, the plantation system would become the impetus for continued exploitation, while European diseases would greatly contribute to Native extinction.

European diseases rivaled the effects of cruelty and oppression. New World Natives encountered by Columbus had been isolated from the microbe population carried by the Europeans. As a consequence, they had very little immunity to these diseases. Syphilis, measles, tuberculosis, smallpox, and the like were devastating to the Native peoples; Amerindians expired quickly from this unexpected biological attack. No doubt, the stress of European oppression and the disruption to traditional food sources also lowered the ability of Native peoples to resist European diseases. By the 1540s, scores of islands in the Caribbean had been completely depopulated, and millions of Native peoples had died as a result of the European onslaught. By 1600, the indigenous Caribbean peoples had essentially perished.[21]

The combined destruction of Native humanity and labor and the rise of sugar production ultimately resulted in the Spanish turning toward African peoples. The Portuguese had already established effective methods for extracting Africans from West Africa and became the principal suppliers of conscript labor. Spain had been unsuccessful in challenging the Portuguese monopoly over the African trade. Columbus planted sugar in the Caribbean in 1493, and by 1522, the island of Hispaniola was exporting sugar.[22] European settlers wanted to expand sugar production, and due to Native extinction, labor was in short supply. A Catholic priest who had come to the New World, Bartoleme de Las Casas, expressed his humanitarian concern for the rapidly disappearing Native population by suggesting that Africans be used to supply the necessary labor for these plantations. The Spanish Crown consented, and by the middle of the century, New World slavery was confined to Africans.[23]

The Africans seemed able to resist European diseases much better than the Native peoples.[24] It is likely that West African maritime and trans-Saharan commerce contributed to substantial long-distance trade. As a consequence, the resulting forms of social intercourse introduced a much broader and diverse body of diseases into the region from an early period. West African immune systems and forms of social organization had had a better opportunity to adapt and fortify themselves against the types of microorganisms carried by Europeans.[25] In the sixteenth century, Africa

remained a viable productive medium for human labor, where the West
Indies was not. Just as the land in the Caribbean was cleared for the
plantations (its cash-crop factories), it also was cleared of its indigenous
human resources, while Africa remained the center of production for human labor. However, the observation that the Spanish based their use of
African labor on the belief that Africans were tough is only part of the
story. What also is essential is the fact that an African labor supply seemed
unlimited in the face of an increasing demand for labor and a dwindling
Native population. The population of enslaved Africans, despite its high
mortality, was refueled by a large West African reservoir of humans.

THE RAVAGES OF ENSLAVEMENT

Despite the ruggedness of the West Africans, we cannot underestimate
the effects of the ravages of enslavement on their health. Once massive
slave trading and the resulting tribal warfare took hold in West Africa,
the ecologies of health declined rapidly. Firearms made warfare more devastating. The gun is what gave Europeans superiority in enslaving Africans, but its introduction into Africa, which led to altering the balance of
power between neighboring peoples and increasing the destructiveness
and frequency of warfare, is what accelerated the slave trade. Once the
need for guns was established, the practice of trading guns only for slaves
was devastating.[26]

Other challenges became endemic to the trade. The strong alcoholic
drinks introduced by the Europeans helped to weaken the Africans physically and militarily.[27] The captured Africans then were made to undergo
a long march (sometimes hundreds of miles) to the coast, where they
would be stored in holding pens called barracoons.[28] Slaves languished in
the holds of ships as they were moved from slave factory to slave factory
to secure sufficient cargo before making the voyage to the West Indies.[29]
Because of stress, injury, thirst, poor sanitation, malnutrition, and the like,
outbreaks of cholera and other deadly diseases often decimated enslaved
Africans in the barracoons as well as aboard ship. As historian John Blassingame explained: "The foul and poisonous air of the hold, extreme heat,
men lying for hours in their own defecation, with blood and mucous covering the floor, caused a great deal of sickness."[30] Traders were typically
concerned with whether they should overpack their ships with slaves to
account for those who would die or carry less slaves in the hope that more
would survive.[31]

Misery was both physical and psychological for the enslaved Africans.
Clearly, malnutrition was likely prior to embarking on the slave ship because of the forced march and the period of confinement in the barracoons. Aboard ship, malnutrition and related maladies stimulated the
onset and heightened the severity of parasitic and contagious diseases, and

they also precipitated severe depressive states.[32] The slave auction brought further mental, physical, and spiritual challenges, as it was extraordinarily degrading and usually included an intimate examination of the genitalia, teeth, skin, and other body parts, as well as branding with a hot iron. These violations of personal body space compounded the shock of separation from friends, family, and community.[33] Furthermore, throughout the enslavement process, African women suffered all too frequently the indignity of sexual exploitation at the hands of their European captors, who most certainly spread venereal diseases to African women. Frazier observed, for example, that "since European males have been the forerunners in the conquest and settlement of areas inhabited by non-European peoples, the spread of venereal disease has been an inevitable consequence of initial race and culture contacts."[34]

Seasoning, the process of breaking in newly arrived slaves in the Caribbean (which could last for several years), was extraordinarily harsh but was symptomatic of the fact that slavery in this environment was principally an economic institution with few humanistic qualities. Traders distributed new arrivals to veteran slaves and specially designated Europeans whose job was to mold novice captives into compliant workers. The slaves literally could be worked to death, and owners gave little attention to reproduction and family life. Absentee landlordism also contributed to a lack of concern for conditions on the islands. Traders tended to overpopulate the islands with slaves, and they seasoned newcomers for reexport and to replenish slave populations, which lacked the ability to reproduce themselves. Additionally, the punishments for insubordination, attempted escape, striking a European, and uprisings were quite severe. Flogging, branding with a hot iron, breaking bones, public mutilation, and death were liberally used to punish and to discourage resistance. There was no fine or imprisonment if an owner killed his slaves. Laws (Black Codes) that regulated the movements and actions of slaves also were a part of the assorted methods of slave control.[35]

The population of Africans in the Caribbean did not increase naturally, but that of Africans in North America did. One explanation is that the North American slave had better protein.[36] Nutrition was, no doubt, important, but nutrition and its relationship to population growth must be understood in the context of the intersection between the organization and character of work and the sex ratio. When there were many fewer women than men, this tended to restrain fertility, but an excess of males could also be indicative of an industrial organization of work that required masculine labor, reducing the opportunity for association between the sexes.[37]

The distinction between gang labor and peasant labor is important to reveal how social organization affected slave health. Gang labor tended to be masculine, less rewarding, more dedicated to a single type of production, and less supportive of family life, as men slept in large barracks. Mines, sugar mills, and some large estates utilized gang labor. The peasant system involved a wider range of activities and a more diverse community, with work completed on a quota system. Once this quota was achieved, workers were free to perform other activities that could be conducive to their well-being, for example, the cultivation of a more diverse food supply. Because under this system of work planters were more likely to purchase equal numbers of males and females, the peasant system provided greater opportunity for community and family life.

The importance of increased worker autonomy in relationship to health is consistent with the observation that emancipation quickly brought natural population increases in the Caribbean. Moreover, even though in general, Latin and Caribbean slave populations grew slower than North American ones, variations in population growth within the former support the finding that differential fertility is related to type of work, labor conditions, and nutrition. The stages of production of a type of plantation system could also be important as this could further define the character and organization of work.[38] The sex ratio (number of males for every 100 females) is important only with regard to its specific relationship to the productive system. For example, more extreme excesses of women relative to men could reverse the fertility-repressing character of various restrictive modes of work.[39]

Despite the health-depressing effects of slavery, the West Africans proved to be exceptionally resilient and capable workers. Their agricultural skills and knowledge of diverse forms of crop production further contributed to their value to the European plantation system and served as an important dimension of their health-promoting survival skills.[40] West African health and curative practices, religious and spiritual beliefs, and communal values also helped enslaved Africans to transcend dehumanization and negotiate profound disruptions to their ecologies of health.[41] Moreover, we should recognize that West Africa presented a formidable environment, which the Europeans could not readily penetrate for any extended period of time. As a consequence, West African adaptive responses and resilience in the New World were, in all likelihood, strengthened by their knowledge of how to negotiate West Africa's environment and its challenges to health. Thus, a critical component to the balance of health is the cultural capital that Africans brought with them.

ECOLOGICAL INVERSIONS TO HEALTH

Using Frazier's conceptualization that "the ecological basis of race relations is concerned with the manner in which the relations of men to their environment determine relationship patterns which developed between men with different racial and cultural backgrounds," we can say that European ventures to extract wealth from various environments that brought them into contact with non-European groups spawned a negative ecology of race relations.[42] Further, this ecological basis of race relations adversely affected African health. Thus, in contrast to a symbiotic relationship, where interactions between organisms may or may not be beneficial, there was the creation of antibiosis, whereby the association between organisms was injurious to one.

Antibiosis became a problem for the Native Americans as well. As Frazier correctly observed, the Native peoples seemed to receive Europeans without fear or hostility. They greeted the Europeans as they would greet any honored guest, with "ceremony and religious significance."[43] However, in every case, the Native peoples were divested of their land and enslaved or exterminated. Furthermore, Frazier revealed the process of European ecological inversion as global in nature, in that biological conflict, changes in plant and animal life, and the destruction of traditional forms of social organization occurred in diverse areas (North America, South America, Central America, New Zealand, Australia, South Africa, and the West Indies) where the Europeans developed settler colonies.

Religion, in general, failed to mitigate European cruelty and, in fact, became a justification for it. Frazier observed that both the British and the Spanish treated the Native Americans with unrestrained brutality and, for example, "In New England the Puritans justified their barbarous treatment of the Indians by appealing to the example of the Hebrews of the Old Testament."[44] European settler colonies characteristically invoked divine providence as the justification for genocidal acts. Thus, religion became a profound cognitive tool for deciding that others were not worthy of respect as humans. Europeans typically saw non-Europeans as having either no religion or a defective one. As a consequence, they constructed bizarre and complex theories of racial supremacy, using biblical sophistry.[45]

As we have already noted, the plantation system had grave implications for non-European peoples. It became the justification for a massive slave trade and introduced brutal and destructive forms of mass labor. The plantation system was also broadly destructive to the environment. It was responsible for extensive soil erosion and the widespread production and distribution of such crops as sugar and tobacco. These specific crops were to become destructive, not only because of the way in which they were produced, but also because of their ensuing mass consumption and deleterious consequences to health. When the Europeans altered traditional patterns of land management and cultivation to implement their cash-crop–oriented systems, the resulting patterns of soil erosion contributed to increased hunger among the Native peoples. Moreover, European modes of cash-crop production tended to reduce the diversity of foods available to the non-European peoples, and they harmfully altered their traditional family life and forms of social authority and order.[46] The jux-taposing of African development with European economic expansion pro-duced an inverse ecological relationship, as European prosperity brought African degradation. This relationship extended to other non-European groups as well.

A major challenge to African-American health is to alter institutional and residual elements of this inverse ecological relationship. Eurocentric scholarship frequently fails to acknowledge the deep implications of these ecological inversions to the past and the current status of African-American health. This myopia is partially determined by the erroneous belief, which had its roots in European theories of racial supremacy, that chattel slavery and other forms of European domination at least were superior to the conditions under which the Africans had had to live prior to European contact. This is the idea that, despite the human toll of op-pression and exploitation, Europeans always brought "progress" and "civ-ilization." The health of West Africans prior to European enslavement is one such issue.

THE NUTRITION QUESTION

It is unlikely that the African population base, which fueled a massive slave trade for 400 years, providing laborers who were more resistant to certain diseases than the Native Americans and Europeans and a human-ity that could survive the rigors of capture, the exhausting march to the coast, the harsh confinement of the barracoons, the stark challenges of the middle passage, the brutality of seasoning, and the degrading realities of slave labor, was habitually weak and malnourished prior to European con-tact. Furthermore, there is no question that the Africans brought various ailments with them to the New World and that Africa had a tremendous array of dangerous diseases that could challenge human existence. The fact of the matter is, however, that the Europeans had great difficulty penetrating West Africa and negotiating its challenges to health, yet the West Africans flourished in this environment. Thus, we should not under-estimate two facts. The first is that the disruptive effects of slavery lowered African resistance and made the West Africans more susceptible to extant disease vectors as well as to those new microbes carried by Europeans. The second is that the health-promoting nutritional base of West African societies was severely and injuriously modified by European enslavement.

Contrary to these judgments, some researchers have argued that the West Africans—despite a preponderance of evidence that newly enslaved Africans and Africans born in captivity were poorly nourished on the plan-tations—were better nourished in slavery than they were before capture and that nineteenth-century slaves were probably better nourished than Africans of the mid-twentieth century.[47] These conclusions are based on arguments that West African diets were confined to a few low-protein, vegetable foods; that bovine milk was rarely consumed; and that animal protein was not available. There is also the feeling that certain West African food taboos restricted nutrition. These researchers also point to research that indicates that Caribbean-born slaves were taller than newly imported slaves.[48]

The argument that West Africans were generally malnourished prior to European enslavement is speculative at best. The onus of this view is based on more current nutritional problems facing West Africa. However, to argue that the region has not changed in 400 years is to grossly underestimate the impact of the slave trade and colonialism, not to mention natural changes to the environment and other crucial mutations. Today it is generally understood that animal protein and bovine milk are not essential for human growth and health. In fact, in this country there is now greater encouragement to consume less animal protein and more vegetable protein. Moreover, most of the world depends on vegetable protein sources. The belief in the consumption of red meat is ethnocentric. If vegetable-protein–consuming cultures are malnourished, it is not because of the protein source, but because of economic, political, and social conditions that affect food production and distribution.[49]

There is also the problem of definition and the failure to address the broader dimensions of nutrition. What does one mean by malnutrition? Food production and consumption that can sustain life, effectively aid the body to resist disease, and provide the conditions for a sense of well-being hardly can be said to be characterized by bad nutrition. Moreover, nutrition is very much related to how foods are produced, prepared, combined, and consumed. African cultures, like other cultures, combine their foods in distinctive ways. Incomplete vegetable proteins—those protein sources that do not provide the essential amino acids that are required (not produced) by the body—may be combined with other vegetable proteins or small amounts of animal protein to provide high-quality, complete protein. The resilience and vitality of enslaved West Africans and their example as a durable workforce suggest that the West Africans had a solid nutritional base prior to bondage.[50]

Many scholars understand, however, the devastating effects that slavery and colonialism have had on the nutrition and health of large regions of Africa. E. Franklin Frazier observed:

In Africa, widespread malnutrition among the natives has resulted from European contact. One of the primary causes of malnutrition has been the driving of the natives from their lands and their confinement to areas inadequate for their needs. . . . European contact has also affected the dietary habits of African peoples by destroying their traditional social organization which provided the labor and system of cultivation necessary for securing a proper diet.[51]

Other researchers of African health acknowledge that "colonial rule had a profound impact on the health of Africans and, indeed, has largely created the continent's present disease environment."[52] Historical imbalances in power—which means Western domination—permit one nation to dictate to another what it will cultivate; "the present world agricultural division of labor which assigns the poor to producing food and raw materials for export to the rich is a hangover from the colonial period."[53]

Solid historical research indicates that wide regions of West Africa enjoyed ample and diverse food sources and a high standard of living. One scholar revealed that eye-witness accounts indicate that around the headwaters of the Congo River, for example, the people were very self-sufficient prior to encountering Portuguese slave trading and were amply supplied with manioc flour, millet, maize, large haricot beans, small beans, round beans, fruit, bananas, sugar cane, yams, gourds, ground nuts, and much fish from nearby rivers.[54] Diverse trading (including trans-Saharan) provided for diverse food sources and a relatively good standard of living.[55] Arab sources indicated that medieval Africa had a very diverse food supply, including a wide array of fruits, vegetables, grains, cattle, fish, vegetable and animal fats, and even milk consumption (more frequently in the form of sour milk).[56]

The various forms of social organization also ensured food production and sharing that would lessen the potential for famine and nutritional deprivation. One scholar observed:

Crops and other goods were distributed on the basis of kinship ties. If a man's crops were destroyed by some sudden calamity, relatives in his own village helped him. If the whole community was in distress, people moved to live with their kinsmen in another area where food was not scarce. In Akan country [Ghana], the clan system was highly organised, so that a man from Brong could visit Fante many hundreds of miles away and receive food and hospitality from a complete stranger who happened to be of his own clan.[57]

Prior to European contact, in the Western Sudan the principal activity of the population was agriculture. The people had domesticated several species of millet and rice. Other groups who lived in open savannah country specialized in cattle production and other domesticated animals, and still others, near the Niger River, were specialists in fishing.[58] Most important, various people adapted food production to the peculiarities of their particular environment and used advanced methods of agriculture, which included terracing, crop rotation, green manuring, mixed farming, and regulated swamp farming.[59] Research indicates that African "agriculture was based on a correct evaluation of the soil potential, which was not as great as initially appears from the heavy vegetation; and when the colonialist started upsetting the thin top-soil the result was disastrous."[60]

The testimony of enslaved Africans also suggest that West Africa was not a place where people typically were malnourished and unhealthy. The slave narrative of Olaudah Equiano, also known as Gustavus Vassa, gives some insight into the agriculture, diet, and general health of West Africans during the period of the slave trade. Olaudah was kidnapped as a boy from his home in what is now the Benin province of Nigeria. He was eventually sold to British slavers in 1756. Olaudah observed:

Bullocks, goats, and poultry, supply the greatest part of [native] food. These constitute likewise the principal wealth of the country, and the chief articles of its commerce. The flesh is usually stewed in a pan. To make it savory we sometimes use also pepper and other spices; and we have salt made of wood ashes. Our vegetables are mostly plantains, eadas [Taro], yams, beans, and Indian corn. . . . Before we taste food, we always wash our hands; indeed our cleanliness on all occasions is extreme; but on this it is an indispensable ceremony.[61]

Olaudah also mentioned that his people drank palm wine but that he had never observed drunkenness. From the same tree that furnished the palm wine the people obtained nuts and oil. Building homes was a communal activity, and people built separate domiciles for sleeping and day activities. The distinctive way in which West Africans had adapted to their environment was exemplified by Olaudah's comment that his people made a special preparation to repel insects. He further explained:

Our land is uncommonly rich and fruitful, and produces all kinds of vegetables in great abundance. . . . Everyone contributes something to the common stock; and, as we are unacquainted with idleness, we have no beggars. The benefits of such a mode of living are obvious. . . . Those benefits are felt by us in the general healthiness of the people, and in their vigour and activity; I might have added too in their comeliness. Deformity is indeed unknown amongst us[:] I mean that of shape. . . . Cheerfulness and affability are two of the leading characteristics of our nation.[62]

After being seized by slave raiders at approximately the age of 12, Sālih Bilāli, a Muslim, who was also known as Tom, became the head driver of Hopeton Plantation in Georgia in 1816. He had been purchased from the Bahama Islands 16 years earlier. Bilāli was born about 1770 at Kianah on the Niger River near the present town of Mopti. Bilāli described his land:

The natives cultivate the soil, and keep large droves of horses, cows, sheep, goats, and some asses. The great grain is rice. . . . Besides rice, they cultivate a species of red maize, millet and Guinea corn. They also grow beans, pumpkins, okra, tomatoes, cucumbers and cotton. They have cocoa-nuts, pine-apples and small yellow figs, which grow on very large trees.
      The usual food is rice, milk, butter, fish, beef and mutton. The domesticated animals are horses, used for riding, asses and camels for carrying loads; cattle, the

bulls of which have lumps on their shoulders, for milk, and meat—sheep, with very long wool, for food and wool—goats and poultry, and dogs for guards. They have no hogs.[63]

Other nineteenth-century narratives suggest that some West Africans had very long average life spans, with some elders living to around 100.[64]

European disruption of Africa's traditional forms of social organization and food production has had grave effects on the nutrition and health of African peoples. In sum, European environmental adaptations (their quest for wealth) produced antagonistic race relations and an inverse ecology of health for African peoples and other non-European groups. Antibiosis, a relationship whereby the association between organisms is injurious to one of them, emerged as a characteristic circumstance. The slave experience, however, produced additional challenges to health on a day-to-day basis, which we will explore in the next chapter.

NOTES

1. E. Franklin Frazier, *Race and Culture Contacts in the Modern World* (Boston: Beacon Press, 1957), p. 92.

2. See Barrington Moore, Jr., *Social Origins of Dictatorship and Democracy: Lord and Peasant in the Making of the Modern World* (Boston: Beacon Press, 1966), pp. 111–155.

3. See the discussions in Sidney M. Wilhelm, "Can Marxism Explain America's Racism?" *Social Problems* 28 (December 1980): 107; and Bart Landry, *The New Black Middle Class* (Berkeley and Los Angeles: University of California Press, 1987).

4. Frazier, *Race and Culture Contacts in the Modern World,* p. 6.

5. See St. Clair Drake, *Black Folk Here and There: An Essay in History and Anthropology,* vol. 2 (Los Angeles: University of California, Center for Afro-American Studies, 1990); and Frazier, *Race and Culture Contacts in the Modern World,* p. 6.

6. Drake, *Black Folk Here and There,* p. 232.

7. Ibid.

8. Ibid., p. 228.

9. Ibid., p. 232.

10. Ibid., p. 234.

11. Ibid.

12. See D. T. Niane, ed., *General History of Africa. Vol. 4, Africa from the Twelfth to the Sixteenth Century* (Paris and London: United Nations Educational, Scientific, and Cultural Organization and Heineman Educational Books, 1984), p. 99; and J. C. deGraft-Johnson, *African Glory: The Story of Vanished Negro Civilizations* (Baltimore, Md.: Black Classic Press, 1986), p. 126.

13. Niane, *General History of Africa,* p. 99.

14. Vincent Bakpetu Thompson, *The Making of the African Diaspora in the Americas, 1441–1900* (New York: Longman, 1987), p. 78.

15. Ibid.

16. Ibid., p. 79.

17. See Jan Carew, "Columbus and the Origins of Racism in the Americas: Part Two" *Race and Class* 30 (July–September 1988): 38, 53; John Duffy, *The Healers: A History of American Medicine* (Chicago: University of Illinois Press, 1979), p. 2.

18. Frazier, *Race and Culture Contacts in the Modern World,* p. 47.

19. Carew, "Columbus and the Origins of Racism in the Americas: Part Two," p. 34.

20. Thompson, *The Making of the African Diaspora in the Americas: 1441–1900,* p. 12.

21. Frazier, *Race and Culture Contacts in the Modern World,* p. 64; Carew, "Columbus and the Origins of Racism in the Americas: Part Two," p. 38; Kenneth F. Kiple, *The Caribbean Slave: A Biological History* (New York: Cambridge University Press, 1984), pp. 9–10; Michael L. Conniff and Thomas J. Davis, *Africans in the Americas: A History of the Black Diaspora* (New York: St. Martin's Press, 1994), pp. 68, 74; David Henige, "On the Contact Population of Hispaniola: History as Higher Mathematics," in Hilary Beckles and Verene Shepherd, eds., *Caribbean Slave Society and Economy* (New York: New Press, 1991), p. 7; Duffy, *The Healers,* p. 5.

22. Drake, *Black Folk Here and There,* p. 236; Michael L. Conniff and Thomas J. Davis, *Africans in the Americas: A History of the Black Diaspora,* pp. 71, 76.

23. Drake, *Black Folk Here and There,* p. 236; John Hope Franklin and Alfred A. Moss, Jr., *From Slavery to Freedom: A History of Negro Americans,* 6th ed. (New York: McGraw-Hill, 1988), pp. 32–33.

24. Kiple, *The Caribbean Slave: A Biological History,* p. 12.

25. See Gerald W. Hartwig and K. David Patterson, eds., *Disease in African History: An Introductory Survey and Case Studies* (Durham, N.C.: Duke University Press, 1978), pp. 8, 10.

26. Basil Davidson, *The African Slave Trade: Precolonial History 1450–1850* (Boston: Little, Brown and Company, 1961), pp. 238–246. The use of the gun was carried to its logical conclusion in colonial Africa with the invention of the machine gun. Europeans initially ignored the potential of this weapon in their wars against each other. However, they readily embraced the machine gun when they found themselves outnumbered by African soldiers who resisted European exploitation and domination. See John Ellis, *The Social History of the Machine Gun* (New York: Pantheon, 1975), pp. 18, 79–102.

27. Thompson, *The Making of the African Diaspora in the Americas: 1441–1900,* p. 87; Frazier, *Race and Culture Contacts in the Modern World,* p. 67.

28. John Blassingame, *The Slave Community,* rev. ed. (New York: Oxford University Press, 1979), p. 6.

29. Kiple, *The Caribbean Slave: A Biological History,* p. 59.

30. Ibid., p. 7.

31. John Hope Franklin and Alfred A. Moss, Jr., *From Slavery to Freedom: A History of Negro Americans,* pp. 36–37.

32. Kiple, *The Caribbean Slave: A Biological History,* pp. 63–65.

33. See Blassingame, *The Slave Community,* pp. 3–20; deGraft-Johnson, *African Glory,* p. 155.

34. Frazier, *Race and Culture Contacts in the Modern World,* pp. 65–66.

35. Franklin and Moss, *From Slavery to Freedom: A History of the Negro Americans,* pp. 43–45.

36. Kiple, *The Caribbean Slave,* pp. 118–119.

37. E. Franklin Frazier, *The Negro Family in the United States,* rev. ed. (Chicago: University of Chicago Press, 1966), pp. 17–18.

38. Humphrey E. Lamur, "Demographic Performance of Two Slave Populations of the Dutch Speaking Caribbean," in Hilary Beckles and Verene Shepherd, eds., *Caribbean Slave Society and Economy* (New York: New Press, 1991), p. 218.

39. Barry W. Higman, "The Slave Populations of the British Caribbean: Some Nineteenth Century Variations," in Hilary Beckles and Verene Shepherd, eds., *Caribbean Slave Society and Economy* (New York: New Press, 1991), p. 224.

40. See Sterling Stuckey, *Going through the Storm: The Influence of African American Art in History* (New York: Oxford University Press, 1994), pp. 40–41.

41. See Hartwig and Patterson, *Disease in African History,* p. 10; and Stuckey, *Going through the Storm,* pp. 40–41.

42. Frazier, *Race and Culture Contacts in the Modern World,* p. 92.

43. Ibid., pp. 41–42.

44. Ibid., p. 48.

45. See, for example, Winthrop Jordan, *White over Black: American Attitudes toward the Negro 1550–1812* (Baltimore, Md.: Penguin Books, 1969), pp. 17–18, 79; and George Fredrickson, *The Black Image in the White Mind: The Debate on Afro-American Character and Destiny 1817–1914* (New York: Harper and Row, 1971), pp. 72–73, 75, 79, 87–88, 102–103.

46. Frazier, *Race and Culture Contacts in the Modern World,* pp. 54–60.

47. See Kiple, *The Caribbean Slave,* pp. 24–25; and Kenneth F. Kiple and Virginia H. Kiple, "Deficiency Diseases in the Caribbean," in Hilary Beckles and Verene Shepherd, eds., *Caribbean Slave Society and Economy* (New York: New Press, 1991), pp. 173–174.

48. Kiple, pp. 24–25; Kiple and Kiple, pp. 173–174.

49. See for example, Susan George, *How the Other Half Dies: The Real Reasons for World Hunger* (Montclair, N.J.: Allanheld, Osmun and Co., 1977); and Alan Berg, *The Nutrition Factor: Its Role in National Development* (Washington D.C.: Brookings Institution, 1973).

50. See Hartwig and Patterson, *Disease in African History,* p. 10.

51. Frazier, *Race and Culture Contacts in the Modern World,* p. 72.

52. Hartwig and Patterson, *Disease in African History,* p. 11.

53. George, *How the Other Half Dies: The Real Reasons for World Hunger,* p. 16; see also Basil Davidson, *Modern Africa: A Social and Political History,* 2d ed. (New York: Longman, 1989), pp. 19–21.

54. Davidson, *The African Slave Trade: Pre-Colonial History 1450–1850,* pp. 155–156.

55. Niane, *General History of Africa,* pp. 1–14, 177, 202–204.

56. See Tadeuz Lewicki, *West African Food in the Middle Ages: According to Arabic Sources* (New York: Cambridge University Press, 1974).

57. Walter Rodney, *How Europe Underdeveloped Africa* (Dar es Salaam, Tanzania: Tanzania Publishing House, 1972), p. 44.

58. Ibid., p. 67.

59. Ibid., p. 48.

60. Ibid.

61. G. I. Jones, "Olaudah Equiano of the Niger Ibo," in Philip Curtin, ed., *Africa Remembered: Narratives by West Africans from the Era of the Slave Trade* (Madison: University of Wisconsin Press, 1967), p. 73.

62. Ibid., pp. 75–76.

63. Ivor Wilks, "Sālih Bilāli of Massina," in Philip Curtin, ed., *Africa Remembered: Narratives by West Africans from the Era of the Slave Trade* (Madison: University of Wisconsin Press, 1967), p. 150.

64. P. C. Loyd, "Osifekunde of Ijebu," in Philip Curtin, ed., *Africa Remembered: Narratives by West Africans from the Era of the Slave Trade* (Madison: University of Wisconsin Press, 1967), pp. 256–266.

3

Antebellum Life and Health

Medical therapy, diagnostic procedures, public health techniques, and nutritional science were not highly developed during the antebellum period, and Blacks and Whites alike suffered from low standards of health and health care. However, the evolving system of White supremacy presented unique challenges to enslaved Africans and their descendants that Whites did not experience. The day-to-day realities of plantation life in the South and the social conditions that subordinated all people of African descent created added burdens that taxed African-American health beyond the normal health-related threats of the day.

THE HEALTH HAZARDS OF SLAVE LABOR

The purpose of African slavery was to provide a cheap and reliable (captive, malleable, and unending) source of labor for European systems of production, both large and small. Long, hard, tedious, and dangerous work was the norm. The health hazards of slave work were provided by farm animals, farm and industrial tools and machinery, the extremes of the weather, and punishment associated with the drive to produce. Savitt, an important observer of slave health, painted a vivid picture of the perils of plantation life. He noted that brucellosis, leptospirosis, and anthrax were examples of diseases found among farm animals that were passed to enslaved Africans.[1]

Brucellosis, a disease of goats, cattle, and pigs, could infect humans through direct contact between skin, wounds, and infected carcasses. Hog-killing time increased the exposure to this disease, as did the slaughter of beef. In humans this infectious disease is called undulant or Malta fever and is characterized by swelling of the joints and spleen, excessive per-spiration, weakness and anemia, and recurrent attacks of fever.[2]

Leptospirosis (mud fever) is another fever-inducing infection of domes-tic animals, which could be spread by contact between the *leptospira* or-ganism found in the animal's urine and the wounds, skin, nose, or mouth of humans. Food and water could also become contaminated with this organism. Rice and sugar fields, swamps, and muddy pastures provided ample opportunity for infection.[3]

Anthrax, which is caused by a bacterium that usually attacks sheep, cattle, horses, and goats, can cause skin pustules, fever, vomiting, diarrhea, and general malaise in humans. Slaves contracted the disease through han-dling animal hides and hair and eating infected meat.[4] The disease could be fatal.

Accidents and environmental hazards were ever-present features of daily life. Slaves usually were not protected from unsafe equipment and machinery. Limbs could be caught in farm machines and require ampu-tation. Injuries to eyes sometimes produced blindness, and burns, scalds, cuts, and falls were common. Accidents involved overturned carts, and there were runaway wagons. Cold weather produced frostbite, and the long hot days brought sunstroke. Tobacco factories, for example, were characterized by unbearable heat, and blisteringly hot conditions in the fields could be exacerbated by swarms of insects (poorly treated insect bites could become festering sores) and poor or insufficient drinking water. Tobacco dust produced lung disease and irritated eyes; the juice produced rashes, and sometimes there was nicotine poisoning. Coal mining brought methane gas explosions, black lung disease, suffocation from lack of ox-ygen, drownings in mine shafts, and flash fires.[5]

Lead poisoning was a significant problem for West African slaves in the early West Indian societies. A major source of lead poisoning came from the rum they produced (lead was used in the distillation machinery). Slaves were more likely to consume new rum that had not been aged, which was more potent alcoholically and more contaminated with lead. House pain-ters also faced a high risk of poisoning from lead paint.[6]

Women and men were subject to comparable work-related health haz-ards and frequently performed similar work. However, there was some sex-ual division of labor. Very few women served as skilled artisans. They usually were not carpenters, coopers, wheelwrights, tanners, blacksmiths, or shoemakers. Women performed such other skilled jobs as cooking, clean-ing, childcare, ironing, spinning thread, weaving, and sewing. Men usually cleared the land of trees, chopped and hauled wood, and rolled logs, but women also could be called on to do this type of work. Women and men worked side by side in the fields, and harvest time usually brought 16-hour days. Women could have the added burden of pregnancy.[7]

Punishment for inadequate production and other violations of slave propriety were significant health hazards. Punishment for women by overseers could merge into a sadistic lust that brought with it sexual abuse.[8] White male fear of African male sexuality made castration an optional form of retribution.[9] However, the amputation and mutilation of ears and feet, as well as whipping, were more general forms of punishment.[10] Historian John Blassingame observed:

Quite frequently, even the most cultured of planters were so inured to brutality that they thought little about the punishment meted out to slaves. Floggings of 50 to 75 lashes were not uncommon. On numerous occasions planters branded, stabbed, tarred and feathered, burned, shackled, tortured, maimed, crippled, mutilated, and castrated their slaves. Thousands of slaves were flogged so severely that they were permanently scarred.[11]

SANITATION, DISEASE, AND EPIDEMICS

The context of slave health often was shaped by poor sanitary conditions and overcrowding that added to the virulence, frequency, and character of the disease environment and a host of life-threatening maladies, including seasonal ailments and epidemics of various kinds. Slaves tended to live in quarters some distance from their owners. Through his research, W.E.B. Du Bois observed that even though slave dwellings varied by the size and location of the plantation and by the plantation's method of management, they shared the common characteristics of sparseness and routine lack of comfort. Du Bois remarked, "the rules and exactions of the plantation favored unhealthy habits."[12] Poor ventilation, lack of windows for sunshine, and damp earthen floors contributed to the growth of fungus and bacteria and to generally stale and stagnant conditions. The slaves themselves complained that cabins were uncomfortable and overcrowded, and two families typically occupied one cabin. Moreover, many slaves lived in sheds, not cabins. Overcrowding contributed to increased contagion. Thus, individual health problems could quickly become serious public health issues.[13]

Even though, as historian John Blassingame revealed, West Africans and Native peoples introduced the daily bath to Europeans, there frequently was a lack of opportunity for personal and public hygiene for the slaves. Unwashed clothes and unclean beds promoted bedbugs and body lice. Often there were not adequate and safe methods for the disposal of waste, which included human excrement and decaying food.[14] Contaminated water, worm- and larvae-infested soil, and rodents contributed to a dangerous public-health environment.[15] Coughing, sneezing, and unclean hands helped to spread disease in a crowded living environment, and a lack of shoes increased the vulnerability to skin penetration by harmful organisms and parasites.[16]

A particularly common and pervasive health problem negotiated by slaves was parasitic worms. Deaths from parasites were high, and, unlike other types of ailments, they were year-round afflictions.[17] Savitt identified five common varieties of intestinal worms afflicting enslaved Africans: the long roundworm (*Ascaris*), the long threadworm (*Trichuris,* or maw worm), the short threadworm, and the broad (fish) and narrow (pork and beef) tapeworms. Because of its size (four to five inches), the *Ascaris lumbricoides* was the most frequently found. Damp soil aided the growth of *Ascaris* eggs in the feces of infected persons. Tapeworms were the second most common parasite and were ingested from poorly cooked or raw, infected meat or fish.[18] Another significant parasite was the hookworm. However, hookworm larvae did not enter humans through the mouth but rather through penetration of the skin—usually bare feet that traversed ground contaminated by the feces of infected humans. Savitt described the characteristics of this malady:

Symptoms included itching . . . as larvae penetrated the skin, transient pneumonia or bronchitis during larval migration through the pulmonary tract, and severe anemia associated with the destruction of red blood cells by the adult worm attached to intestinal mucosa. . . . Chronic sickness was the lot of those infected, accompanied by an enormous appetite, retarded mental, physical, and sexual growth among children, extreme lethargy, generalized edema . . . and chronic leg ulcers.[19]

In addition, dirt eating, or geophagy (a practice continued from West Africa), facilitated ingesting infected soil.[20]

Most types of diseases experienced by enslaved Africans were seasonal. Intestinal diseases characterized the summer months and respiratory ones the winter months.[21] Certain epidemics like yellow fever also were dependent on warm weather, as the disease-carrying *Aëdes aegypti* mosquito has a short life span and fails to bite in cool weather.[22] Generally speaking, respiratory secretions helped to spread a host of infections during the winter months, and disease-causing microorganisms proliferated in warm, moist environments. The crucial factors were poor sanitation, crowding, poor ventilation, and poor nutrition, which lowered resistance to disease. Cancer and diseases of the heart and circulatory system did not appear to be major causes of slave deaths because infectious diseases ended lives before significant numbers of people reached the age to contract these degenerative ailments.[23] However, it is reasonable to assume that many of these ailments went undiagnosed.

One historian of slave health observed that the most dreaded epidemics of the antebellum period were cholera and yellow fever.[24] However, typhoid and other epidemics also created considerable concern. Domestic and endemic diseases like malaria, smallpox, dysentery, scarlet fever, influenza, and pneumonia could reach epidemic proportions. Port cities were particularly susceptible to epidemics and were usually the location of cholera and yellow fever outbreaks.[25] Cities increased the conditions for contagion, and ports heightened the opportunity for the entry of new human disease vectors. West Africans were less susceptible to yellow fever than Europeans, but significant numbers did contract the disease and die from it. Yellow fever is a viral disease that is native to Africa, and some Africans had become resistant to the disease from surviving an earlier bout with the affliction in their youth.

Cholera caused many more African than European deaths. It is a bacterial disease transmitted through food and water and is particularly troublesome in areas with poor sanitation. Moreover, the intense work requirements of slaves meant greater consumption of water, which was often contaminated. Slaves also suffered from nutritional deficiencies that made them less capable of recovering from an attack of cholera.[26]

Smallpox, influenza, pneumonia, and dysentery caused many deaths annually among enslaved Africans and, though endemic, often reached epidemic proportions. Smallpox is a viral disease, and transmission is from human to human rather than from mosquito to human, as in yellow fever. Effective vaccinations were used in this hemisphere by the early 1800s, but many enslaved Africans remained unvaccinated. As a consequence, smallpox epidemics continued to kill many slaves. Smallpox is endemic to Europe, but by the 1800s, it had been present in Africa for centuries. Ironically, many Africans had learned to immunize themselves through a technique that Europeans later called variolation. The European minister-physician Cotton Mather heard of this technique from his African slave and promoted it in eighteenth-century colonial America.[27] Influenza epidemics killed many enslaved Africans, but pneumonia was the more fatal of the respiratory ailments, a class of diseases that seemed to kill more Blacks than Whites.[28] Dysentery or "bloody flux" was frequently fatal and was transmitted through contaminated fecal matter. Flies and unsanitary conditions helped spread the disease. Bloody stools characterized the malady; epidemics were common and annually incapacitated the slaves for days and even weeks.[29]

Among the most common endemic diseases that challenged the daily lives of antebellum Africans in America was malaria. Africans and Europeans brought malaria with them to the New World, and methods of clearing the land that left reservoirs of stagnant water served to proliferate the breeding places of infected mosquitoes.[30] Malaria is an acute and sometimes chronic infectious disease caused by the invasion of protozoan parasites within red blood cells. The disease is spread through infected female anopheles mosquitoes, which pass the parasites on to humans through their bites:

If the anopheles mosquito was not already available in North America to spread the malarial parasite, it was exported from England and Holland; the open water caskets and water buckets on sailing vessels and the presence of infected passengers and crew would have facilitated the passage.[31]

As was the case for yellow fever, Europeans observed and were amazed that Africans had greater resistance to malaria than they themselves. Proportionately speaking, Africans died less often and contracted milder cases. Malaria was no insignificant disease for the Africans, however. They could survive and function better than the Europeans or Native Americans under the ravages of malaria, continuing to perform the backbreaking work of European plantations, but malaria nonetheless caused the Africans much misery and death on a regular basis. Of the four types of malaria, *Plasmodium vivax, Plasmodium falciparum, Plasmodium malariae,* and *Plasmodium ovale,* the first three were of relevance to New World Africans.[32] *P. vivax* is the most widespread globally, while *P. malariae* is found in many parts of the world but is most prevalent in Africa. These varieties caused fewer deaths. *P. falciparum* is more deadly and is responsible for the most deaths in Africa and other tropical regions.[33]

West Africa's intense encounter with malaria produced certain immunologic and adaptive responses to the disease. Various blood anomolies found among West Africans and people of West African descent tend to resist certain forms of malaria. Examples are sickle-shaped blood cells and the glucose 6-phosphate dehydrogenase (G6PD) deficiency trait. These traits and their variants tend to resist the multiplication of malarial parasites in *P. falciparum* malaria.[34] There also seems to be a relative resistance of West Africans and some unexposed African Americans to *P. vivax* malaria, which is presumably associated with a common deficiency trait among West Africans whereby they possess red blood cells that lack the Duffy group antigen determinants, Fy^a and Fy^b.[35] The Duffy group is one type of blood group system. Blood groups are distinguished by the antigens located on mature red blood cells and are genetically determined. Antigens induce the formation of antibodies and form the basis of immunity.

Other deadly and harsh endemic diseases include consumption (tuberculosis), dropsy, tetanus, and the complications of pregnancy. Tuberculosis is more deadly to virgin populations, and since Africa had little exposure to this essentially European disease, it was much more destructive to Blacks than Whites under similar environmental conditions.[36] Dropsy (edema), the generalized condition in which the body retains an excessive amount of tissue fluid and appears enormously bloated, was much more common among enslaved Africans than Whites.[37] Tetanus, an extremely painful infection that is usually fatal, often entered the dirty wounds of slaves and caused excruciating deaths at a much higher rate than in Whites. Tetanus is caused by an anaerobic bacterium that commonly lives in the intestines of horses. The spores live in soil and dust and produce a deadly toxin when they enter wounds and multiply. The hazards of work and unsanitary conditions made tetanus a particular concern for slaves.[38]

Pregnancy and birth were dangerous events, which took the lives of enslaved African women and their newborns more frequently than Whites. Neonatal tetanus, the result of an infected umbilical cord, was particularly troublesome for enslaved Africans and greatly contributed to high rates of infant mortality. An important cause of maternal mortality was puerperal fever which, like neonatal tetanus, was precipitated by deliveries done under unsanitary conditions.[39] Nutritional deficiencies made pelvic deformities a characteristic problem for slave women, requiring taking the life of either the mother or the newborn. This problem made cesarean sections particularly important. Some enslaved African women brought the knowledge of this technique with them. However, in North America, White physicians perfected their use of this operation by experimenting on slave women.[40]

Venereal diseases seemed to be less of a problem among antebellum Blacks than Whites.[41] There was no evidence of epidemics like the ones that occurred in Europe, and the Africans themselves saw syphilis and gonorrhea as White diseases.[42] However, we should recognize that the spread of venereal diseases among enslaved Africans was significantly connected to the system of exploitation and oppression. Transmission was from European men, who had little reason to control their lust for African women. Numerous testimonies by slaves indicated that White males (overseers and planters) sexually pursued slave women relentlessly and that sexual favors were usually obtained by force.[43]

Yaws, an African disease, is caused by an organism similar to the syphilis spirochete but is not venereal. However, in the antebellum South, yaws was at times mistaken for syphilis. An extremely ugly disease, it is characterized by benign, fleshy tumors and raspberry-like open ulcers covering large portions of the body; it is not fatal. Yaws tended to protect against syphilis, but the disease died out by the Civil War. After this time, syphilis became more of a problem for African Americans. The isolation of the plantation and the strong commitment to family life had helped to contain syphilis.[44] Greater mobility after the war, limited exposure to venereal diseases, continued sexual exploitation by White males, ignorance regarding transmission of the diseases, and inadequate methods of treatment would make venereal diseases much more problematic for African Americans in the postbellum period.

FOOD, NUTRITION, AND HEALTH

The diet of enslaved Africans was a tremendously important determinant of their health. It affected their ability to resist infectious diseases and to recover from illness and injury. The rigors of daily toil and the stress, strain, and pain of enslavement added to the nutritional requirements of slave workers. Arguments that the average food allotted to slaves exceeded modern caloric and nutritional requirements have proven to be misstated. In fact, the slave diet was dangerously deficient. There were problems of nutritional imbalance, poor-quality food, underfeeding, and lack of variety. Slave owners had little knowledge of nutritional requirements and balance; however, their own diets were considerably more diverse and of better quality.[45]

As a rule, enslaved Africans had a greater chance of elevating their health status with increased control of their own food production, preparation, and consumption. However, the ecology of race relations militated against such controls. Cash crops in the South competed with food crops, and food selection for slaves was inextricably linked to the agricultural objectives, whims, and penuriousness of the slave owners.[46]

Because it was inexpensive to produce and easy to preserve, pork became the preferred protein source of southern Whites, who commonly also issued the meat to slaves. The planters, however, gave slaves the worst or fatty cuts and took the better or leaner cuts for themselves. A ration of cornmeal typically complemented the pork diet. Owners claimed that cornmeal and fat pork were particularly appropriate for enslaved Africans because of "heat-producing properties," which made them valuable "muscle-producing foods."[47]

The fat pork–cornmeal diet became the nutritional foundation for slave culture and was usually sporadically and inadequately supplemented with other foods. For the majority of adult slaves, a peck of corn and three or four pounds of salt pork or bacon was the weekly allowance, and on some plantations, slaves never consumed fresh meat, milk, eggs, or fruit and rarely had vegetables.[48] Some slaves received beef or mutton on special occasions, but this was infrequent. Slave owners supplemented daily rations of corn and pork with sweet potatoes, vegetables, fruits, and, occasionally, molasses, salt, and coffee.[49] Planters rarely gave whiskey to slaves but found that the slaves could be made more content if they were allowed to chew, sniff, and smoke tobacco.[50]

For their own consumption, slaves produced turnips, sweet potatoes, cowpeas (black-eyed peas), cabbage, collards, pumpkins, onions, okra, and squash. Some slaves owned poultry and hogs, but they frequently sold their vegetable and animal produce to acquire other needed items or to save money to purchase their freedom.[51] This made these foods unavailable, to any great extent, to boost slave nutrition. Milk production and consumption was low and was usually in the form of buttermilk. Whole milk and butter were rare, and cheese was almost never consumed.[52]

Rice and wheat were the most commonly consumed secondary grains.[53] Wheat was consumed in bread, cakes, and pancakes but, like that used by Whites, it was unenriched, processed flour without germ or bran and was less nutritious than cornmeal.[54] When possible, slaves also foraged, hunted, and fished for food, and they ate fruits and melons when in season.[55]

Food preparation and processing had varying health implications. Methods of preserving pork involved large amounts of salt, which has proven to be very detrimental to Black health.[56] Southern Blacks and Whites tended to overcook vegetables. Typically, Southerners boiled greens and other vegetables in large pots for hours with fat pork or bacon. For greens, the resulting liquid, called "pot-likker," was thrown away by Whites but consumed by Blacks, usually mixed with crumpled cornbread.[57] The liquid, of course, contained the important nutrients of the vegetable. Blacks did not prepare vegetables haphazardly, however, and allowed for different cooking times as they added various ingredients to a dish. Perhaps influenced by the dearth of cooking utensils, multiple foods were boiled and prepared in large metal pots.[58] Because Africans cooked for themselves and Whites, African foods (for example, rice, sorghum, watermelon, okra, peanuts, sesame seed, and black-eyed peas) and spices heavily shaped southern cooking and tastes, even though food selection was limited by the conditions of enslavement.[59] Genovese observed:

The slave cooks established their reputation, to no small degree, by their imaginative spicing. The subtle flavors of the gumbos and jambalayas . . . arose primarily from black skill in combining herbs. Sesame seeds and oil, as well as red pepper, came from Africa with the slaves and became central to southern cooking.[60]

Methods of cooking varied. Sometimes individual families would cook for themselves, but there also were communal or common kitchens.[61] Planters found that common kitchens gave them better control over food supplies and made more field hands available.[62] In some cases children had to compete for a finite quantity of food at a given time from a common trough, literally eating like pigs.[63] Toward the end of the antebellum period, communal cooking was preferred but was not used everywhere.[64]

Food shortages, lack of variety, and poorly balanced diets were common and contributed to an array of health problems for the enslaved Africans. Scholars have observed that slaves commonly revealed through their autobiographies that they had had at least one owner who did not give them enough food. Moreover, provisions could run low regardless of the propensity of the slave owner, and food shortages of meat, wheat flour, sweet potatoes, cowpeas, and green and yellow vegetables were common.[65] Inadequate quantities of rations and lack of variety motivated many slaves to steal food.[66]

The slave diet, even if high in caloric content, was low in protein and important vitamins and minerals. As a consequence, hunger could remain high despite the consumption of large amounts of food. Hunger was highest and nutritional deficiency diseases most prevalent when vegetable consumption was lowest, usually during the winter months. Thus, the slave culture that emerged was built around a poorly balanced and nutritionally deficient diet of fat (pork), sweets (syrups and molasses), and cereals (usually corn but also, to a lesser degree, processed wheat and rice). Finally, a high proportion of slaves had to contend with parasitic worms at some time during their lives. Intestinal worms shared the slaves' nutrition and interfered with the normal utilization of such nutrients as protein, vitamins A, C, and B12, and iron.[67]

The symptoms of various diseases were similar, and it is hard to identify nutritional deficiency diseases from antebellum medical descriptions. However, solid evidence suggests that beriberi, from a deficiency of the B vitamin thiamine, and pellagra, from a deficiency of the B vitamin niacin, were a normal part of slave life.[68] Furthermore, the high-carbohydrate and high-fat diets increased the need for B vitamins, and their short supply strongly suggests that many slaves were unable to properly metabolize carbohydrates, fats, and proteins.[69]

Other deficiencies were likely among the slave population. Vitamin C, a nutrient that is needed on a daily basis, was consumed erratically, and deficits were linked to the seasonal unavailability of fresh fruits and vegetables. Vitamin A shortages were similarly linked to the undersupply of green and yellow vegetables, as well as to consumption of poor-quality vegetables. Deficiencies in iron and vitamin B12 contributed to anemia, and deficiencies in calcium, magnesium, and vitamin D contributed to such diseases as rickets and tetany.[70]

Nutritional deficiencies severely affected the quality of life of the enslaved Africans and made daily labor even more challenging. Beriberi produced fatigue, diarrhea, appetite loss, poor memory, sleep disturbances, disturbed nerve function and paralysis, wasting of limbs, weight loss, edema, and heart failure in adults, and convulsions, respiratory difficulties and such problems as nausea, vomiting, constipation, diarrhea, and abdominal discomfort in afflicted infants. Pellagra produced fatigue and weakness, diarrhea, loss of appetite, weight loss, reddened and swollen tongue, depression and anxiety, disorientation, impairment of memory, and dermatitis. Severe deficiencies of vitamin C resulted in scurvy, but less severe deficits caused, among other symptoms, impaired digestion and utilization of iron, poor lactation, bleeding gums, and lowered resistance to infection. Vitamin A deficiencies especially affected the eyes and skin. Night blindness, the inability to adjust to darkness, was one of the first symptoms. Blotchy skin, loss of the sense of smell, loss of appetite, fatigue, corneal ulcers, and soft bones and teeth were other symptoms. Anemia brought, among other problems, a general weakness, and tetany, a children's disease, included symptoms of convulsions and spasms of the voluntary muscles.[71]

OPPRESSION, STRESS, AND HEALTH

Poor nutrition lowered the resistance of the enslaved Africans to infectious diseases, but the role of stress in the disease process has generally been overlooked by researchers in their discussions of slave health. Stressors are forces acting on the body that move it away from some equilibrium state, and stress is the nonspecific result of any demand on the body. These demands exceed the body's adaptive resources and contribute to lowered resistance to disease, premature aging, and early death.[72]

Physical or environmental, social, and psychological stresses are the three types that humans must address. Environmental stress may involve extremes of heat and cold and levels of toxicity. Social stress involves events that disrupt groups through death, divorce, rapid social change, the exigencies of poverty, and the like. Psychological stress involves addressing individual feelings of fear, anxiety, worry, panic, inferiority, frustration, anger, and others. Some feel that psychological stressors are more intense because of their more enduring character.[73]

The critical process is the stress or arousal response. This response consists of physiological and psychological reactions to stimuli or stressors. There is a release of adrenal hormones that stimulate the "fight-or-flight," emergency response. Blood pressure is raised, depth of breathing increases, sweating occurs, and the large external muscles contract. If stress is prolonged, insulin production is inhibited and there is sodium and water retention.[74] The stress arousal response especially depletes the B complex vitamins and vitamins A and C. It interferes with the absorption of calcium, potassium, zinc, copper, and magnesium. Besides its effects on the nutritional integrity of the body, prolonged stress tends to suppress the immune system and disrupt its efficiency. In fact, it is likely that all disease is stress related because of the effect of stress on the immune system.[75]

For the enslaved Africans, prolonged stress must have been a strikingly important aspect of daily life. The breakup of the slave family was common, and the threat of sale was a routine method of social control. Such familial disruptions were, no doubt, intensely anxiety producing.[76] The uncertainty of new owners and a new environment added to the distress of separation.[77] Overcrowding in the slave quarters was another source of stress. The fact that enslaved Africans lacked control over intimate aspects of their lives was demoralizing and frustrating. Owner controls over food, clothing, shelter, family life, sexual practices, and medical care were examples. Moreover, in order to demean them, owners typically ignored the names of their slaves and called them what they wanted. White male sexual abuse of African wives and daughters and the practice of concubinage had to have been particularly stressful.[78] Masters and overseers sought to instill in slaves a sense of inferiority and obsequiousness, and they used a diverse system of rewards and punishments to divide the slave community in order to bring about conformity and control. Owners and their agents sought to shatter Black unity and trust by using Blacks to hurt other Blacks.[79]

The sources of intense stressors related to oppression seemed endless. Slaves who lost their usefulness as workers could be disposed of by being sold to hospitals and medical schools.[80] The requirements of survival, which created the need to internalize aggression and, at times, redirect aggression at innocent loved ones, produced additional stress for individual slaves and the slave community in general.[81] The demands of performing multiple tasks on the plantation often became overwhelming. Women, for example, frequently had to care for children while performing time-consuming, arduous, and backbreaking work in the fields.[82] The strain of having to maintain a split personality—one for the master and one for the slave community—was great.[83] High mortality and the resulting problem of bereavement also took its toll.[84] In short, tremendous uncertainty and upheaval, anxiety, recurrent disruptions to family life, the physical stress of punishment, sadism and brutality, toxic conditions (poor sanitation), constant loss of status, and routine intrusions into their intimate and personal space heightened stress for the slave population far beyond what one could consider normal.

The slave diet without question was inadequate to help mitigate the nutritional effects of stress or fortify the body against extraordinary and prolonged stress. The nutrients that were routinely lacking in the diets of bondsmen and -women were exactly those that were depleted even more by the typical conditions of physical, social, and psychological stress. Deficiencies in the B-complex vitamins must have been especially problematic. The high-sugar and -starch diets of the slaves increased the need for these nutrients. Excessive stress particularly depletes the B vitamins, and we have already noted the high probability that many slaves suffered from certain vitamin B–deficiency diseases like beriberi and pellagra. The stress of oppression did not end with slavery but continued as racial oppression took on new forms. The rural and urban experiences continued to exemplify an ecology of race relations that subverted African-American health.

NOTES

1. Todd L. Savitt, *Medicine and Slavery: The Diseases and Health Care of Blacks in Antebellum Virginia* (Chicago: University of Illinois Press, 1978), p. 105.

2. Ibid.

3. Ibid.

4. Ibid.

5. Ibid., pp. 106–109; Richard B. Sheridan, *Doctors and Slaves: A Medical and Demographic History of Slavery in the British West Indies, 1680–1834* (Cambridge: Cambridge University Press, 1985), pp. 189–190; Anne S. Lee and Everett S. Lee, "The Health of Slaves and the Health of Freedmen: A Savannah Study," *Phylon* 38 (1977): 177.

6. See Jerome S. Handler, Arthur C. Aufderheide, Robert S. Corruccini, Elizabeth M. Brandon, and Lorentz E. Wittmers, Jr., "Lead Contact and Poisoning in Barbados Slaves: Historical, Chemical, and Biological Evidence," in Kenneth F. Kiple, ed., *The African Exchange: Toward a Biological History of Black People* (Durham, N.C.: Duke University Press, 1987), pp. 140–157, 160.

7. Jacqueline Jones, *Labor of Love, Labor of Sorrow: Black Women, Work and the Family, From Slavery to the Present* (New York: Vintage Books, 1986), pp. 16–18, 23, 27.

8. Ibid., pp. 20, 33.

9. Winthrop Jordan, *White over Black: American Attitudes toward the Negro 1550–1812* (Baltimore, Md.: Penguin Books, 1969), pp. 154–159.

10. See Sheridan, *Doctors and Slaves,* pp. 179–182, 190.

11. John W. Blassingame, *The Slave Community,* rev. ed. (New York: Oxford University Press, 1979), pp. 262–263.

12. W.E.B. Du Bois, ed., *The American Family,* The Atlanta University Publications, no. 13 (Atlanta, Ga.: Atlanta University Press, 1908), p. 48.

13. Savitt, *Medicine and Slavery,* pp. 50–51; Blassingame, *The Slave Community,* p. 254.

14. Blassingame, *The Slave Community,* p. 101; Savitt, *Medicine and Slavery,* pp. 51, 58–62.

15. Savitt, *Medicine and Slavery,* p. 51.

16. Ibid., pp. 51, 61.

17. Ibid., p. 63.

18. Ibid., pp. 64–66.

19. Ibid., p. 70.

20. See Kenneth F. Kiple and Virginia H. King, *Another Dimension to the Black Diaspora: Diet, Disease, and Racism* (New York: Cambridge University Press, 1981), p. 74; Savitt, *Medicine and Slavery,* p. 66.

21. Savitt, *Medicine and Slavery,* pp. 51, 58.

22. Kiple and King, *Another Dimension to the Black Diaspora,* p. 32.

23. Lee and Lee, "The Health of Slaves and the Health of Freedmen," p. 176.

24. William D. Postell, *The Health of Slaves on Southern Plantations* (Gloucester, Mass.: Peter Smith, 1970), p. 5.

25. Lee and Lee, "The Health of Slaves and the Health of Freedmen," p. 172.

26. Ibid., pp. 173–174; Kiple and King, *Another Dimension to the Black Diaspora,* p. 156.

27. John Duffy, *The Healers: A History of American Medicine* (Chicago: University of Illinois Press, 1979), pp. 35–36; Kiple, *The Caribbean Slave,* pp. 144–145; Lee and Lee, "The Health of Slaves and the Health of Freedmen," p. 173.

28. Savitt, *Medicine and Slavery,* p. 53; Postell, *The Health of Slaves on Southern*

Plantations, p. 81; Kenneth F. Kiple, *The Caribbean Slave: A Biological History* (New York: Cambridge University Press, 1984), p. 144.

29. Savitt, *Medicine and Slavery*, pp. 62–63.

30. Postell, *The Health of Slaves on Southern Plantations*, p. 7.

31. Duffy, *The Healers*, p. 11.

32. Kiple, *The Caribbean Slave*, p. 14.

33. Ibid.; see also Richard A. Williams, ed., *Textbook of Black-Related Diseases* (New York: McGraw-Hill, 1975), pp. 449–452.

34. Ibid., pp. 210–214; Kiple, *The Caribbean Slave*, p. 15.

35. For a more extended discussion see Kiple, *The Caribbean Slave*, pp. 15–17, 21.

36. Kiple and King, *Another Dimension to the Black Diaspora*, pp. 139–146.

37. Lee and Lee, "The Health of Slaves and the Health of Freedmen," p. 175; Kiple and King, *Another Dimension to the Black Diaspora*, p. 145.

38. Lee and Lee, "The Health of Slaves and the Health of Freedmen," p. 175.

39. Ibid., pp. 175–178; Savitt, *The Health of Slaves*, pp. 117–120.

40. See Herbert M. Morais, *The History of the Negro in Medicine* (New York: Publishers Company, 1967), p. 12; Duffy, *The Healers*, pp. 140–143.

41. Eugene Genovese, *Roll Jordan Roll: The World the Slaves Made* (New York: Vintage Books: 1976), p. 459.

42. Ibid., pp. 459–460; Kiple, *The Caribbean Slave*, pp. 243–244.

43. Blassingame, *The Slave Community*, p. 154.

44. Postell, *The Health of Slaves on Southern Plantations*, pp. 80–81; Blassingame, *The Slave Community*, p. 171.

45. Kiple and King, *Another Dimension to the Black Diaspora*, pp. 79–80; Kenneth M. Stampp, *The Peculiar Institution: Slavery in the Ante-Bellum South* (New York: Vintage Books, 1956), pp. 282–283; Sam B. Hilliard, *Hog Meat and Hoecake: Food Supply in the Old South, 1840–1860* (Carbondale: Southern Illinois University Press, 1972), p. 62.

46. See Hilliard, *Hog Meat and Hoecake*, p. 27.

47. Stampp, *The Peculiar Institution*, p. 283; Hilliard, *Hog Meat and Hoecake*, p. 42.

48. Stampp, *The Peculiar Institution*, pp. 282, 284–285.

49. Hilliard, *Hog Meat and Hoecake*, pp. 56, 59.

50. Genovese, *Roll Jordan Roll*, p. 644.

51. Savitt, *Medicine and Slavery*, pp. 95–96.

52. Hilliard, *Hog Meat and Hoecake*, p. 62.

53. Ibid., p. 50.

54. Savitt, *Medicine and Slavery*, p. 94.

55. Hilliard, *Hog Meat and Hoecake*, pp. 51, 56.

56. Kiple and King, *Another Dimension to the Black Diaspora*, p. 199.

57. See Genovese, *Roll Jordan Roll*, p. 548; Hilliard, *Hog Meat and Hoecake*, p. 51.

58. Hilliard, *Hog Meat and Hoecake*, p. 62.

59. See Blassingame, *The Slave Community*, pp. 39, 103.

60. Genovese, *Roll Jordan Roll*, p. 542.

61. Ibid., p. 544.

62. Hilliard, *Hog Meat and Hoecake*, p. 62.

63. Genovese, *Roll Jordan Roll,* p. 507.

64. Hilliard, *Hog Meat and Hoecake,* p. 62; Postell, *The Health of Slaves on Southern Plantations,* p. 37.

65. Hilliard, *Hog Meat and Hoecake,* pp. 63–64; Savitt, *Medicine and Slavery,* p. 89; Kiple and King, *Another Dimension to the Black Diaspora,* pp. 85–87.

66. See Blassingame, *The Slave Community,* p. 254; Genovese, *Roll Jordan Roll,* pp. 603–604.

67. Savitt, *Medicine and Slavery,* p. 89.

68. Ibid., pp. 87–88; Kiple and King, *Another Dimension to the Black Diaspora,* pp. 124–128.

69. Kiple and King, *Another Dimension to the Black Diaspora,* p. 91.

70. Kiple and King have argued that deficiencies of calcium were common among enslaved Africans and were exacerbated by a high incidence of lactose intolerance and dark skin. Lactose intolerance made milk an unlikely option to obtain calcium, and dark skin does not synthesize vitamin D as efficiently as light skin. Vitamin D is necessary for the effective absorption of calcium. See Kiple and King, *Another Dimension to the Black Diaspora,* pp. 89–94, 96–106; and Savitt, *Medicine and Slavery,* pp. 89–93; see also Nutrition Search, Inc., *Nutrition Almanac,* rev. ed. (New York: McGraw-Hill, 1979), pp. 64–65, 110, 160–161.

71. Symptoms for these deficiencies are widely known. See Nutrition Search, Inc., *Nutrition Almanac,* pp. 15, 44, 110, 117, 156–157; Kiple and King, *Another Dimension to the Black Diaspora,* pp. 89–90, 101–104, 122–128; and Kiple, *The Caribbean Slave,* pp. 82–85, 89–103.

72. See Jonathan C. Smith, *Understanding Stress and Coping* (New York: Macmillan, 1993), pp. 6–8.

73. Donald R. Morse and Robert L. Pollack, *Nutrition, Stress, and Aging: A Holistic Approach to the Relationship among Stress and Food Selection, Digestion, Nutrients, Body Weight, Disease, and Longevity* (New York: AMS Press, 1988), pp. 1–2.

74. Ibid., pp. 3–5.

75. See Smith, *Understanding Stress and Coping,* pp. 117–130; Morse and Pollack, *Nutrition, Stress, and Aging,* pp. 10–11; Dorothy H. G. Cotton, *Stress Management: An Integrated Approach to Therapy* (New York: Brunner/Mazel, 1990), p. 175.

76. See, for example, Norrece T. Jones, Jr., *Born a Child of Freedom, Yet a Slave: Mechanisms of Control and Strategies of Resistance in Antebellum South Carolina* (Hanover, N.H. and London: University Press of New England, 1990), p. 63; Blassingame, *The Slave Community,* pp. 173–177.

77. Blassingame, *The Slave Community,* p. 290.

78. Ibid., pp. 154–155, 183.

79. Jones, *Born a Child of Freedom,* pp. 90, 98–100, 105–106.

80. Ibid., p. 122.

81. Ibid., p. 206; Blassingame, *The Slave Community,* p. 225.

82. Blassingame, *The Slave Community,* pp. 180–181.

83. Ibid., pp. 205, 304.

84. Ibid., p. 177.

4

The Challenges of Post-Slavery Rural and Urban Life

The fundamental relations of race that contributed to a negative ecology of health for African Americans remained unchanged in the post-slavery period. European initiatives to dominate and exploit new lands using African labor had already transformed institutional and cultural processes among Africans in America in such a way that their status became tied to the vagaries of European American economic designs. African lives were also subject to harsh realities and stressful uncertainties stimulated by wide variations in European racialist thinking. This thinking was largely couched in religious ideology but was expressed later in pseudoscientific theories that were intended to make inferior Africans and people of African descent. This is not to say that African-American lives were totally controlled by White enclaves of power and their subordinates; however, the tendency to perpetuate powerlessness and dependency among Blacks as a class was routine and pervasive.

THE BEGINNING OF ECONOMIC DISLOCATION

Chattel slavery connected African lives to European American economic goals, but emancipation brought new forms of misery and increasing economic dislocation. For African Americans, the later part of the nineteenth century brought distinctively new challenges because of the way in which White elites sought to extract wealth from the environment. The political, economic, and cultural interests of emerging industrial elites in the Northeast were to clash with the political, economic, and cultural interests of a southern, landowning aristocracy. The result was a civil war that marked triumphant movement toward dominance by an industrial economy over an agricultural one. At this point, the need for African labor would begin a pivotal transformation, and the plantocracy, with its cash-crop system, would begin to fail, largely because of the exhaustion of the soil and the changing market conditions for cotton.

White supremacy reemerged in new and virulent forms to shape the character of economic competition. As a consequence, White racism systematically excluded African Americans from gaining a solid connection to the emerging industrial economy as owners and workers. White northern elites did bring African Americans into the industrial workforce on a limited basis, but only when White bodies were inadequate. White land-owning elites in the South continued to try to eke out cash-crop profits (largely from cotton) from their exhausted soil by tying African Americans to the land in abject poverty and degradation. Poor Whites suffered also; however, White supremacy served to subordinate and inferiorize all African Americans and limit their ability to compete equally in all areas of economic activity.[1]

Critical survival-related events for African Americans were the disorganizing experiences of the Civil War, the failure of land reform, and political disenfranchisement following Reconstruction. Emancipation from chattel slavery, although desirable, was a substantial crisis for African Americans because they lacked the essential tools to sustain themselves. The social welfare initiatives of the Freedmen's Bureau were temporary, and efforts to break up large plantations and provide ex-slaves with land to support themselves were short-lived and unsuccessful. Therefore, the masses of African Americans, who were essentially farmers, had to return to their former owners as tenants and sharecroppers, only to find themselves routinely cheated, exploited, and kept dependent and poverty stricken.[2]

Southern Whites took away the political gains achieved by African Americans during the period of the Reconstruction, when White southern and northern elites reached a new political compromise and created a fresh coalition of White supremacy. During Reconstruction, African Americans were used by northern, industrial elites (Republicans) to solidify their domination over the South (Democrats). To do this, African-American males received the right to vote. This meant, of course, increased political leverage for Republican objectives. However, African Americans quickly were sold out when new accommodations were made between White southern and White northern property-owning elites. The Rutherford Hayes–Samuel Tilden election of 1876 signaled the end of this coalition and resulted in the removal of federal troops from the South. This act ended protection for African-American human and citizenship rights for nearly 80 years.[3]

White planters conspired to obtain African-American labor for nothing and, as Carter G. Woodson described:

[Blacks] had no land, no mules, no presses nor cotton gins, and they could not acquire sufficient capital to obtain these things. They were made victims of fraud in signing contracts which they could not understand and had to suffer the consequent privations and want aggravated by robbery and murder by the Ku Klux Klan.[4]

Blacks held the worst and most unhealthy jobs, but had to give them up when White men needed them. In general, African Americans had to relinquish skilled jobs that would pay well. Lerone Bennett observed, for example, that only 20,000 of the 120,000 artisans in the South were White following the Civil War, yet this number was reversed by 1900.[5] This state of affairs was enforced by violence and intimidation. Following the war, for example, Whites typically murdered Blacks in the South for political reasons. Between 1866 and 1879, 3,500 African Americans were killed (this included various massacres), yet no one was ever arrested or brought to trial.[6]

The tenant system in the South formed the foundation for a new slave system. Most large tracts of land remained owned by White planters and were dedicated to cotton production. Black tenant farmers began each year with mortgages that consumed everything they owned, all their labor, and everything they would produce before they had harvested a single crop. African Americans had to pay a third of their product for use of the land, an exorbitant fee for recording the contract, and two to three times as much as they should for ginning their cotton. If any crop was left, it was eaten up by other charges, real or imagined, that the planter placed on the price of goods obtained by the tenant.[7] Landless Blacks were thrown into a criminal and immoral cycle of debt that was protected by a corrupt legal system and a system of racial etiquette that demanded the most abhorrent obsequiousness under the threat of losing one's livelihood or even being lynched. Perhaps the most profound symbol of Black subordination was the ability of many White planters to sexually exploit the wives and daughters of their Black tenants with impunity.[8]

These oppressive conditions precipitated a steady flight by African Americans from the land to new locations which, no doubt, was destabilizing to an infrastructure of health. Propertyless Blacks and property-owning Blacks who lost their possessions were forced to move to southern towns and cities.[9] Moreover, although there had been significant movement through the South by ex-slaves following the Civil War, the first organized migration began in 1879 when thousands of African Americans from Louisiana, Mississippi, Texas, and Alabama began a trek to Kansas, where they hoped to get land, mules, and money from the government. Some Blacks went to other western states; for example, in 1889 and 1890, African Americans sought to settle in the Oklahoma territory. Whites attempted to stop the exodus to Kansas, and White immigrants in Oklahoma met Blacks with racial hatred and mob violence. Nevertheless, many African Americans successfully settled in these two regions. Woodson noted that Native Americans greatly assisted the African-American settlements.[10] In Oklahoma, Blacks formed 25 all-Black communities. These were efforts to build a life free from racial hatred and exploitation and to find economic prosperity.[11]

RURAL COMPLICATIONS

Rural life in the post-slavery period yielded a wide array of health problems for the masses of African Americans. Generally speaking, poor health and disease followed poverty—which meant unsanitary, shoddy, and overcrowded living conditions—and malnutrition. In the Black Belt, cotton competed with food production for personal consumption. This curtailed diversity in the diet. Money to buy food, clothing, and medical services was scarce. Access to emergency medical care was already difficult in isolated rural communities, and racial segregation gave Blacks limited or no access to these services when available. The use of physicians were also time consuming and expensive. Nearly all doctors were White, and some were landowners; neither status brought a feeling of trust or security to oppressed southern Blacks.

An intense system of racial segregation and exploitation continued to provide added stress for African Americans. Lynching, a corrupt legal system, and the threat of losing one's livelihood were the principal methods of enforcing dependency and racial subordination. Illiteracy was another method of control. White landowners discouraged their Black tenants and sharecroppers from securing an education. This made Blacks dependent on the land; they had low expectations, were unable to discern ways to transcend their oppression,[12] and were ignorant of the rules of bookkeeping. However, the greatest problem was that Whites cheated Blacks with impunity.[13]

Blacks experienced significantly poorer health than Whites. Environmentally, overcrowding, inadequate sanitation, malnutrition, and the stress produced by a White supremacy system heightened the conditions promoting disease. Developmentally, constraints on literacy and education hindered self-help efforts among African Americans. This socially induced ignorance made it more difficult to conceive, execute, and institutionalize progressive health-enhancing activities. Thus, the poorer health of African Americans was produced by antibiosis and the resulting problem of underdevelopment.

Maladaptation to antibiosis is the dysfunctional way in which people may adjust to the constraints of exploitation in order to survive. Poor dietary habits that derive from adaptation to limited, inadequate, and nutritionally imbalanced food sources are examples. Adaptive responses are

initially circumstantial and conditional but can become dysfunctional cultural habits. In the context of cultural hegemony, dysfunctional cultural
habits are very difficult to alter because they frequently are reinforced by
the system of exploitation (especially if their continuation is in the interest
of powerful elites) and become tied to the identity of the group, whose
members now view such habits as traditional.

Well into the twentieth century, the vestiges of slavery and the plantation system disadvantageously shaped the lives of African Americans.
Charles S. Johnson's classic study of the deteriorating plantation economy
in Macomb County, Alabama—a region characteristic of the entire Black
Belt of approximately 200 counties and whose population was more than
half African American—illustrated the relationship of White supremacy
and cotton production to the sickness and disease of southern Blacks.[14]
Johnson analyzed 612 rural African-American families in the 1930s. He
observed that there had been no change in farming methods since slavery
and that tenants remained dependent on planters for food, clothing, shelter, small cash advances, and various other staples.[15]

The struggle to live was always enormously challenging, but the struggle
increased as the soil became increasingly exhausted.[16] Pellagra and other
nutritional-deficiency diseases were pervasive.[17] Mothers routinely lost
children in childbirth, and there were high numbers of miscarriages and
stillbirths.[18] People generally did not understand why their children died,
and mothers accepted the deaths of their infant with a dreary fatalism.[19]
Reports of suffering were universal and included accounts of open sores,
uncontrollable fits, tumors, fevers, loss of teeth, excruciating and generalized pain, shortness of breath, digestive disorders, back problems, and
mental malaise.[20] The chief causes of death remained heart disease, stillbirths, tuberculosis, influenza, nephritis, cancer, pellagra, and malaria.[21]

Poor housing and sanitation paralleled an intense struggle with disease
and suffering. Most housing consisted of one- or two-room cabins, and
dwellings were in such poor condition that tenants did not look upon them
as houses. The wall coverings routinely were newspapers, and tenant domiciles generally leaked and barely provided protection against the elements. There was no indoor running water, and only the fortunate had
privies near their abodes. Sanitation was atrocious, and some dwellings
had no sewage disposal at all. Open wells, well pumps, and springs provided water, but some people lacked any source of water.[22]

Diets were nutritionally inadequate and followed the slave culture. The
winter diet was salt meat, corn or flour bread, and syrup or sorghum. Very
few vegetables were eaten. Meals had little variation, and eating was irregular. Breakfast was usually cornbread and syrup, while a heavy meal
with meat was eaten at supper. Fortunate people had potatoes to put away
for the winter. Large numbers of families ate no vegetables in winter or
summer. Some people were able to grow gardens in the summer, but ten-

ants frequently sold those goods for small amounts of cash to buy other staples.[23] The consequence, of course, was widespread malnutrition. These findings were consistent with late nineteenth- and twentieth-century dietary studies of African Americans in the South, whose diets were high in calories but low in protein, iron, calcium, and phosphorus. Vegetable, egg, dairy, and fruit consumption was low, while the consumption of fats, sweets, and cereals was high.[24]

Raper's classic study of Macon and Greene counties in Georgia in the 1920s and 1930s painted a similar picture of antibiosis and dependency. First, he noted that peaceful race relations were dependent upon the norm of White supremacy, which was buttressed by the threat of lynching.[25] Additionally, many African-American families were accustomed to experiencing the nutritional deficiency diseases of rickets and pellagra. Raper observed:

Fresh garden foods, such as carrots, beets, okra, spinach, squash, parsnips, English peas, and lettuce, while affording a considerable proportion of the food of a few, constitute probably less than one-tenth of the food consumed by the mass of rural families. Their diet, rich in fats and low in vitamin content, is one of the main factors accounting for the low vitality, frequent ill health, high susceptibility to contagious disease, and high death rate among farm and tenant families.[26]

Again, the cotton system militated against diversified food production, and tenants were not enthusiastic about growing their own food after working all day for the landlord. African Americans who owned land were better able to grow their own food, have diversified diets, maintain better health, and claim lower infant and maternal mortality.[27] A typical meal for landless farmers was fried fat meat, cornbread and molasses, and coffee with sugar when times were good.[28]

Another negative adaptation of slave culture was the continued reliance upon tobacco as a palliative. The poorest segments of the community consumed the most tobacco. The trade and consumption of tobacco among African Americans was encouraged by the landowners, as planters found that it kept their tenants pacified. Smoking was more of a man's pastime, but you also found women smoking old clay pipes. Men, women, and children all used snuff and chewed tobacco.[29]

URBAN TRENDS

The declining cash-crop system of southern agriculture based on cotton ultimately led to increased African-American urban migration in the South and to the North. Previously, in 1860, there were 4.5 million African Americans, of which 89 percent were slaves, and 90 percent lived in the South. Of this percentage, nearly all lived in rural areas.[30] However, from about 1880, increasing numbers of African Americans migrated to find work and better opportunities in southern towns and cities. Frazier informs us that by 1910, nearly 1.67 million African Americans in the South had migrated from the state where they were born to another state. He argued that most of this migration was to urban areas in the South. Nearly 1 million had moved about the South, and approximately 400,000 had gone North.[31] Between 1890 and 1910, the proportion of African Americans in urban areas increased from 20 to 27 percent, a seemingly small increase but indicative of a trend that would rapidly accelerate in the next several years.[32] In the North, despite the fact that there was no large regional redistribution of the African-American population, such cities as New York, Chicago, and Philadelphia experienced significant increases in the proportions of their African-American populations.[33]

The great stream of northern, urban migration, which was also known as the Great Migration, began in 1915 and was associated with World War I. There were certain push and pull factors that brought African Americans in droves to the North and its urban centers. Several push factors were a depressed demand for labor, low wages, and low cotton prices. In 1915 and 1916, a boll weevil infestation damaged crops in Louisiana, Mississippi, Alabama, Georgia, and Florida. These same states suffered large floods in the summer of 1915. Segregation, discrimination, lynching, poor educational opportunities, a corrupt and racist legal system, and the tenant method of crop production were additional, noteworthy motivations to leave the South.[34] However, these push factors were important but not sufficient to stimulate massive, northern urban migration.

The critical impetus to northern urban migration was the pull factor of jobs and economic opportunity. Before World War I, European immigration was over 1,000,000 a year, but because of the war, it dropped to 326,700 in 1915 and under 200,000 in 1916 and 1917. With World War I curtailing European immigration at a time when industry was expanding, White businesses sought southern Blacks on a limited basis to meet their labor needs.[35] Whites flocked to the better-paying jobs stimulated by the war effort, creating a shortage in common labor.[36]

The trend away from agricultural work to urban-based employment for African Americans expanded dramatically. Racism, however, permitted virtually no development of an African-American business and property-owning class. Blacks, for the most part, were restricted to unskilled labor and, because of the nature of an industrial, wage-based economy, became a growing class of consumers.[37] This result is important because class underdevelopment and dislocation contribute to a cycle of radical dependency and, for African Americans, radical dependency always has contributed to poor health outcomes.

At first, in the late nineteenth century, the mortality of Blacks in urban areas was higher than in rural areas, probably because of the combined problem of overcrowding and poor sanitation. Additionally, many rural migrants brought with them infectious diseases and habits that were ill-suited for urban environments, especially when those environments did not adequately meet a variety of crucial sanitation, housing, and public health needs. Between 1920 and 1940, northern urban mortality dropped below southern rural mortality, but the urban disadvantage still persisted in the South.[38]

The early problem for cities in the late nineteenth and early twentieth centuries was that of managing human waste, as populations became more dense, so as not to contaminate water and food supplies, heighten contagion, and increase the toxicity of the environment. Improved sanitation meant living in a household with a toilet that was connected to a sewer system. It also meant having access to a bathtub.[39] The 1890s seemed to be a turning point in public health measures.[40] Prior to 1850, so-called "heroic" medicine had predominated. White physicians typically bled and purged their patients as treatments for a wide range of ailments.[41] It was not until the latter part of the nineteenth century that scientific research revealed disease vectors in the form of bacteria and other pathological agents. From this period, health officials used sanitary engineering to control contagious diseases.[42]

The general trends in African-American health from the mid-nineteenth to the early twentieth century were reflected in the mortality and life expectancy statistics of the period. They illustrated the added tax of racial oppression and the relationship of antibiosis. Although such statistics are incomplete and unstandardized, best estimates compiled from a variety of sources suggest that between 1850 and 1860, 280 to 320 African-American children per 1,000 died before their fifth birthday. This rate was probably 50 percent higher than the rate for rural White children.[43] From 1850 to 1880, African-American mortality declined only slightly or not at all. Mortality rates were relatively constant between 1880 and 1910, but after 1910, mortality for all ages, especially in urban areas, began to decline. Throughout, however, African-American mortality rates were never close to the lower rates and greater declines for Whites of the same periods. By 1940, African Americans were about 20 years behind Whites in their risk of mortality.[44] Moreover, in 1900, the estimated life expectancy of Blacks was between 33 and 35 years of age, about 16 years less than that of the White population.[45]

Urbanization for African Americans meant battling infectious diseases. Such diseases were sensitive to improvements in sanitation and nutrition, both of which were continuing problems in the light of structured inequality and maladaptations to antibiosis. W.E.B. Du Bois captured these issues in his groundbreaking study of Philadelphia Blacks. He found that African Americans "dwell in the most unhealthful parts of the city and in the worst houses in those parts."[46] Du Bois observed problems with the city's waste disposal system and drinking water and noted that mortality rates among African Americans varied along with the quality of their living conditions. He also found poor dietary habits among African Americans and revealed that poor families could not afford to buy nourishing food because of the cost of rent.[47]

We find a similar picture of environmentally induced health problems facing late nineteenth-century and early twentieth-century African Americans in New York City. In 1890 in New York, 37.5 Blacks per 1,000 died, compared to 28.5 per 1,000 Whites. Between 1895 and 1915, African-American deaths annually exceeded births by around 400. Tuberculosis and pneumonia were consistently the greatest killers of African Americans.[48] In the early 1920s, for example, tuberculosis killed three times more Blacks than Whites in New York City. New York's Harlem (the largest Black community in America) had a mortality rate 42 percent higher than the city rate. Harlem mothers died in childbirth at twice the rate of mothers from other areas. There were excessive deaths from heart disease and cancer and excessive cases of rickets and syphilis. Between 1923 and 1927, Harlem's infant mortality was 111 per 1,000, compared to 64.5 per 1,000 for the entire city.[49]

Osofsky informs us that African-American deaths from tuberculosis were so alarmingly high that a branch of the New York Tuberculosis and Health Association was founded in Harlem in the 1920s. This organization was called the Harlem Tuberculosis and Health Committee. The committee focused on controlling tuberculosis but also addressed other health issues. Nutrition, prenatal care, and social hygiene were several of its concerns. Twelve African-American dentists opened a free clinic, and committee doctors visited homes to locate pretubercular people. The committee delivered public lectures on diet, child care, and the etiology of tuberculosis to churches, fraternal organizations, and schools. It distributed written information on crucial health issues, and children who were particularly malnourished and destitute were sent to the country for fresh air and a nutritious diet. The work of the committee did help to reduce tuberculosis, but everyone involved understood that there had to be a serious attack on the social conditions that spawned infectious and nutritional diseases.[50]

The emergence of New York's Harlem as America's largest African-American community exemplified the growth of Black communities throughout the urban North. As increasing numbers of African Americans fled to urban areas in the pursuit of better opportunities and human freedoms, they were confined to specific locations. Geographical confinement, or ghettos, became the norm. Ghettos were a new tool to control and subordinate African Americans. White absentee ownership of real estate and essential businesses created adverse economic returns since money spent in the African-American community routinely flowed outside it.

Bombings, mob violence, police brutality, restrictive covenants (agreements between realtors not to rent or sell to Blacks), and the like were used by Whites to limit the areas where Blacks could live. As a consequence, African Americans typically were forced into overcrowded conditions and made to pay more for rents, mortgages, insurance, and other goods and services.[51] Segregation may not have been written in law, but it was affirmed by the complicity of dominant institutional arrangements and normative White supremacy.

Chicago developed its African-American ghetto by 1915. People of all classes were compressed in large contiguous neighborhoods. There were variations in the housing stocks, but large sections of the community were slumlike. Discrimination in the job market confined African Americans to the lowest-paying jobs, which Whites did not want. In 1900, nearly 65 percent of Black men and over 80 percent of Black women worked as domestics and in personal services. In 1910, 45 percent of employed Black men worked as porters, servants, waiters, and janitors, and 63 percent of Black women were domestic servants and laundresses.[52] Similarly, in the 1930s, African Americans in Chicago were extremely underrepresented in professional, business, clerical, and skilled and semiskilled jobs, and they were overrepresented in unskilled jobs and domestic and servant work.[53]

In short, wretched social conditions in Chicago produced poor African-American health. In 1925, African-American mortality rates were twice those of Whites, even though Chicago had the lowest death rates of any city of 1,000,000 or over. In the latter part of the 1920s and early 1930s, three Black babies died for every two White babies. For every White homicide, six Blacks were killed. African Americans contracted tuberculosis at 5 times the rate of Whites and venereal diseases at 25 times the rate of Whites. Between 1939 and 1941, Chicago Blacks died from tuberculosis at a higher rate than in any other metropolitan city in the United States.[54]

Drake and Cayton noted that high mortality rates were related to the standard of living and ignorance about infectious diseases and how they were spread. They also pointed out that the absolute number of cases of syphilis and gonorrhea did not warrant the belief that the African-American community was being destroyed by venereal diseases. In 1942, 75 venereal diseases per 1,000 were reported for Blacks and 3 per 1,000 for Whites. Moreover, Blacks had had less exposure to tuberculosis and thus had achieved less immunity. Overcrowding was so great in Chicago for many African-American communities that many of their public schools ran in double and triple shifts.[55] Furthermore, on Chicago's South Side, the African-American population was so congested that in the late 1930s and early 1940s, Blacks lived 90,000 to a square mile, compared to 20,000 persons to a square mile in adjacent White neighborhoods.[56]

Other problems that compounded urban health problems were illegal drug use and a lack of adequate recreational facilities. Henri observed that Whites sold southern rural Blacks cocaine, and the use of that stimulant was increasing in southern cities in the early 1900s. Increased crime was related to illegal drug use; moreover, the drug habits moved North with the migrants.[57] Physical health also suffered from a lack of constructive recreation. Because of segregation, many recreational facilities were restricted to African Americans. Parks, beaches, theaters, dance halls, amusement parks, swimming pools, and the like were not as readily available to Blacks as they were to Whites. Music and dance were the most available recreational activities for African Americans, but White exploitation and control over the venues for these activities often placed even dancing in a distasteful context.[58] African Americans frequently had little control over what went on in their communities, and a White power structure, for example, often placed activities like prostitution, which served largely a White clientele, in Black neighborhoods.[59] Such practices, of course, compounded already the troublesome public health problems in African-American communities.

Urbanization as a general trend continued for African Americans but slowed down during the Depression. The southern economy continued to worsen, but a poor national economy curtailed job opportunities in the North. However, World War II restimulated industrial expansion in the early 1940s, and African-American migration to the northern cities resumed with great intensity. Between 1950 and 1960, every southern state except Florida, Maryland, and Delaware had a net out-migration of its African-American population, and westward movement—primarily to California—reached major proportions (over 300,000) for the first time.[60] By 1940, nearly half of all African Americans lived in urban areas; by 1950, the proportion was 62 percent; in 1960, 73 percent; and in 1970, 81 percent. However, in 1970, 53 percent of the African-American population still lived in the South, 39 percent lived in the North (in 1870, only 9 percent lived in the North), and 9 percent lived in the West (in 1870, the percentage was negligible).[61]

Generally speaking, the second wave of urbanization marked an era of declining deaths from infectious diseases, increasing deaths from degenerative diseases, declining infant and maternal mortality, and an increasing life span. Gone were the times, at the turn of the century, when tuberculosis killed more African American than any other disease. Nevertheless, positive health changes for African Americans continued to lag far behind those for European Americans. For example, deaths from all causes for Black men were 142 percent of the deaths for White men in 1950 and 146 percent in 1983. Deaths from all causes for Black women were 172 percent of the deaths for White women in 1950 and 150 percent in 1983.[62] Furthermore, although deaths from diseases of the heart were very prevalent as well among African Americans early in the twentieth century, they were overshadowed by deaths due to infectious diseases. Later years would be characterized by the increasing prominence of deaths from such degenerative diseases as diabetes, cancer, cirrhosis, and the social disease of homicide.[63]

POST-INDUSTRIALISM: THE MATURING OF ECONOMIC DISLOCATION

The added stress of economic instability, poverty, migration, discrimination, segregation, and White supremacy racism contributed greatly to the health problems suffered by urban African Americans. However, African Americans did not meet these health-related crises passively. Extensive self-help efforts, the struggle for civil and human rights, and a range of other endeavors to stimulate institutional and community development helped to stem the tide of negative external forces. If one carefully scrutinizes the serious and deep character of structured inequality and racism, one can legitimately conclude that African Americans have done amazingly well in the light of so many assaults on their well-being and existence. However, the old challenges persist and new ones abound.

The family was one crucial institution that helped African Americans resist environmental attacks to their health. Billingsley observed that between the end of slavery and World War II, the African-American family was amazingly stable. As late as 1960, 78 percent of all African-American families with children were headed by married couples.[64] This was at a time when over 50 percent of all African Americans lived below the poverty line.[65] In 1990, the number of African-American families with children and headed by married couples declined to 39 percent. Moreover, in 1980, for the first time, female-headed families with children outnumbered married-couple families with children.[66] The decline in double-headed families with children paralleled a decline in the strength and resiliency of the traditional African-American extended family.[67]

The late 1960s and early 1970s marked a turning point for the African-American family. During this period, industrial development as a function of expanding manufacturing jobs had peaked in terms of its effect on enlarging an African-American working class. This working class had been spawned by the earlier phenomena of industrialization, migration, and urbanization, coupled with a limited need for African-American labor. However, I have already noted the tenuousness and fragility of African-American working-class development because of structured inequality and White supremacy racism. African Americans, therefore, were hurt most by the ensuing process of deindustrialization, which involved the loss of manufacturing jobs, and were in the poorest position to compete for service sector, white-collar jobs. Thus, at the time that African Americans became predominantly urban, the manufacturing jobs departed from the urban centers. A steep decline in the stability of the African-American family followed the decline in the African-American working class.[68] This historical turning point was also marked by a reversal of previous migratory trends. For the first time, in the late 1960s and early 1970s, we begin to see a decline in African-American northern migration and increased movement back to the South.[69]

In the post-industrial era, old and new challenges connected to the historical relationship of antibiosis and the maturing of economic dislocation are producing distinctive health-related problems for African Americans. Underground economies (the sale of illegal drugs, etc.) have become more virulent. The stress of being African American and living under a normative White supremacy system persists and, in many cases, has intensified. Deaths from traditional infectious diseased have declined dramatically over the years but, in this day and age, they are still abnormally high. Moreover, social and economic conditions help to spread new infectious diseases like AIDS. Furthermore, the decline in marriage has negative implications for sustaining community health. This is because deaths from degenerative and lifestyle-related diseases are particularly sensitive to the status of the family, as is the ability to manage stress. Consumer manipulation becomes more intense in a post-industrial economy because of the need to exploit existing markets more efficiently, and the family is important to mediate this process effectively.

In the next chapter we will investigate folk, popular, and alternative health practices among African Americans. These practices represent important indigenous efforts to control various factors affecting health. They can help us to understand the cultural basis of health behavior and the difficulties involved in developing appropriate institutional responses to health problems under the conditions of cultural hegemony.

NOTES

1. See, for example, Lerone Bennett, Jr., *Confrontation: Black and White* (Baltimore, Md.: Penguin Books, 1966), pp. 66–93; E. Franklin Frazier, *Black Bourgeoisie: The Rise of a New Middle Class* (New York: Free Press, 1957), pp. 15–19; Frazier, *The Negro Family in the United States,* rev. ed. (Chicago: University of Chicago Press, 1966), pp. 209, 225.

2. Ibid.

3. Ibid.

4. Carter G. Woodson, *A Century of Negro Migration* (New York: Russell and Russell, 1969), p. 128.

5. Bennett, *Confrontation: Black and White,* p. 81.

6. Woodson, *A Century of Negro Migration,* p. 128; Emmett J. Scott, *Negro Migration during the War* (New York: Arno Press and the New York Times, 1969), p. 4.

7. Woodson, *A Century of Negro Migration,* pp. 132–133.

8. See Hortense Powdermaker, *After Freedom: A Cultural Study in the Deep South* (New York: Russell and Russell, 1968), p. 192; Hylan Lewis, *Blackways of Kent* (New Haven, Conn.: College and University Press, 1964), p. 252; Arthur R. Raper, *Preface to Peasantry: A Tale of Two Black Belt Counties* (New York: Atheneum, 1968), p. 72.

9. Woodson, *A Century of Negro Migration,* p. 130.

10. Ibid., pp. 134–138, 143–145; Scott, *Negro Migration during the War,* p. 6; Daniel M. Johnson and Rex R. Campbell, *Black Migration in America: A Social Demographic History* (Durham, N.C.: Duke University Press, 1981), pp. 51–53.

11. Johnson and Campbell, *Black Migration in America,* p. 65.

12. See, for example, Charles S. Johnson, *Shadow of the Plantation* (Chicago: University of Chicago Press, 1966), pp. 129, 136.

13. Ibid., pp. 120–128.

14. Ibid., pp. 16, 207; see also Raper, *Preface to Peasantry,* p. 3.

15. Johnson, *Shadow of the Plantation,* pp. 14–23.

16. Ibid., p. 24.

17. Ibid., pp. 14, 38–39, 42.

18. Ibid., pp. 33–43, 57–60.

19. Ibid., pp. 192–193.

20. Ibid., pp. 194–195.

21. Ibid., p. 187.

22. Ibid., pp. 93–100.

23. Ibid., pp. 36, 101–102, 109–117.

24. Sam B. Hilliard, *Hog Meat and Hoecake: Food Supply in the Old South, 1840–1860* (Carbondale: Southern Illinois University Press, 1972), pp. 66–68.

25. Raper, *Preface to Peasantry,* p. 23.

26. Ibid., p. 52.

27. Ibid., pp. 54, 70.

28. Ibid., p. 43.

29. Ibid.

30. Karl E. Taeuber and Alma F. Taeuber, *Negroes in Cities: Residential Segregation and Neighborhood Change* (New York: Atheneum, 1969), p. 11.

31. Frazier, *The Negro Family in the United States,* pp. 209–210.

32. U.S. Bureau of the Census, *The Social and Economic Status of the Black Population in the United States: An Historical View, 1790–1978,* Current Population Reports, Special Studies Series P-23, no. 80 (Washington, D.C.: U.S. Government Printing Office, 1979), p. 14.

33. Johnson and Campbell, *Black Migration in America,* p. 67.

34. Woodson, *A Century of Negro Migration,* pp. 168–171; Scott, *Negro Migration during the War,* pp. 18–22.

35. See Frazier, *Black Bourgeoisie,* pp. 44–45; Bennett, *Confrontation: Black and White,* pp. 114–115.

36. Scott, *Negro Migration during the War,* pp. 52–53.

37. See Frazier, *Black Bourgeoisie.*

38. African Americans were overwhelmingly rural; see Douglas C. Ewbank, "History of Black Mortality and Health before 1940," in David P. Willis, ed.,

Health Policies and Black Americans (New Brunswick, N.J.: Transaction Publishers, 1989), pp. 107, 126.

39. Ibid., p. 121.

40. Duffy, *The Healers,* pp. 230–231.

41. William D. Postell, *The Health of Slaves on Southern Plantations* (Gloucester, Mass.: Peter Smith, 1970), p. 8.

42. Duffy, *The Healers,* pp. 193–194.

43. Ewbank, "History of Black Mortality and Health before 1940," pp. 100–128.

44. Ibid., pp. 112, 125–126.

45. See U.S. Bureau of the Census, *The Social and Economic Status of the Black Population in the United States,* p. 117.

46. W.E.B. Du Bois, *The Philadelphia Negro: A Social Study* (New York: Schocken Books, 1967), p. 148.

47. Ibid., pp. 161–162.

48. Gilbert Osofsky, *Harlem: The Making of a Ghetto, Negro New York, 1890–1930* (New York: Harper and Row, 1966), pp. 8–9.

49. Ibid., p. 141.

50. Ibid., pp. 152–154.

51. See Florette Henri, *Black Migration: Movement North 1900–1920* (Garden City, N.Y.: Anchor Press/Doubleday, 1975), p. 108; St. Clair Drake and Horace R. Cayton, *Black Metropolis: A Study of Negro Life in a Northern City,* vol. 1, rev. ed. (New York: Harper and Row, 1962), pp. 61–66; Allan H. Spear, *Black Chicago: The Making of a Negro Ghetto, 1890–1920* (Chicago: University of Chicago Press, 1967), pp. 24–25, 201; Osofsky, *Harlem,* p. 140.

52. Spear, *Black Chicago,* pp. 11, 24–25, 29.

53. Drake and Cayton, *Black Metropolis,* p. 230.

54. Ibid., p. 202.

55. Ibid., pp. 202–205.

56. Ibid., p. 204.

57. Henri, *Black Migration,* pp. 110–111.

58. Ibid., pp. 114–115.

59. Spear, *Black Chicago,* p. 25.

60. Taeuber and Taeuber, *Negroes in Cities,* p. 13.

61. U.S. Bureau of the Census, *The Social and Economic Status of the Black Population in the United States,* pp. 13–14.

62. Reynolds Farley and Walter R. Allen, *The Color Line and the Quality of Life in America* (New York: Oxford University Press, 1989), pp. 42–43.

63. See David McBride, *From TB to AIDS: Epidemics among Urban Blacks since 1900* (Albany: State University of New York Press, 1991), p. 10; U.S. Bureau of the Census, *The Social and Economic Status of the Black Population in the United States,* pp. 118, 124.

64. Andrew Billingsley, *Climbing Jacob's Ladder: The Enduring Legacy of African-American Families* (New York: Simon and Schuster, 1992), p. 36.

65. U.S. Bureau of the Census, *The Social and Economic Status of the Black Population in the United States,* p. 49.

66. Billingsley, *Climbing Jacob's Ladder,* p. 37.

67. Ibid., pp. 37–38, 40–41, 51; see also Elmer P. Martin and Joanne Mitchell Martin, *The Black Extended Family* (Chicago: University of Chicago Press, 1978), pp. 83–102.

68. Billingsley, *Climbing Jacob's Ladder,* pp. 137–139.

69. Johnson and Campbell, *Black Migration in America,* p. 170.

5

Folk, Popular, and Alternative
Health Practices

Folk, popular, and alternative health beliefs and practices among African Americans are, to a great extent, the result of the erosion of the institutional basis of West African medical techniques and approaches in the New World, which was caused by the imposition of chattel slavery and European cultural hegemony. Moreover, folk, popular, and alternative medicine among African Americans involves the molding and reshaping of African, Asian, Native American, European, and other available health care methods into distinctive health care traditions that exist parallel to mainstream medicine. These health care practices, as we shall see, have developed a unique coherence and have become connected socially, historically, and conceptually.

The terminologies of folk, popular, and alternative beliefs overlap and roughly point to health care approaches that differ from mainstream orthodox medicine. *Folk medicine* is associated with healing traditions that are not connected to Western orthodox medicine. This terminology may suggest an earlier tradition that is waning or one that embodies older systems of knowledge. *Popular medicine* is a more neutral term and encompasses medical traditions maintained by ethnic or class segments of the society that are distinct from professionals and specialists who engage in Western orthodox medicine.[1]

Alternative medicine is also broadly defined and includes health and healing practices that are intended to replace the drug, surgical, and radiation therapies of orthodox medicine. For example, alternative medicine includes practitioners of *naturalistic* health care systems like naprapathy, colon therapy, naturopathy, acupuncture, and chiropractic, who ideologically do not, and legally cannot, use drugs, surgery, or radiation therapy.

It also includes orthodox medical practitioners who prefer not to use drugs, surgery, or radiation to treat disease. Patients seek alternative medicine in cases where they perceive orthodox medicine as ineffective or harmful.[2]

Alternative medicine typically maintains an expanded view regarding the basis of health, the etiology of disease, and the value of various therapeutic options.[3] Moreover, within this category of health care, we find the roots of people-based movements to reform the limitations, harmful features, and cultural dominance of orthodox medicine. The reform of orthodox medicine has far-reaching social implications since the development of Western medical dominance carries with it connections to patterns of class, race, and gender exploitation.[4] We also should note that folk, popular, and alternative health care systems are differentiated based on their practice by formally and informally trained practitioners (that is, different degrees of institutionalization) and lay persons who utilize such techniques in self-care.

CULTURAL HEGEMONY AND AFRICAN MEDICINE

The problem of cultural hegemony is embodied in the way that African medicine encountered European medicine.[5] African medical practices were as effective or superior to European ones throughout the more than 400 years over which the Europeans forcibly expropriated African labor for their own economic ends.[6] To justify the exploitation of African peoples in the New World under chattel slavery and later, in Africa, under colonialism, the ideology of White supremacy grew to permeate intellectual and popular thought among Continental Europeans and European settler colonies.[7] All things African were deemed inferior by the Europeans, despite a reality to the contrary. African medical practices were strongly integrated with African religious practices, and European religious intolerance contributed to the condemnation of African medical views and techniques. Moreover, African medical techniques had to adapt to severe alterations in their social organization and institutional processes brought about by the conditions of chattel slavery and the requirements of a plantation order.[8]

Cultural repression and delegitimation tended to splinter and distort African health and healing practices in the New World in unknown and diverse ways. Underdevelopment became a problem since there were now barriers to traditional methods of preserving knowledge and training medical practitioners. Thus, in instances where Africans in the New World were able to bring and preserve relevant cultural capital, their medical techniques could be highly adaptive, innovative, and effective. However, in some instances, medical approaches became fragmented, distorted, and retrogressive.

The key issue is that for enslaved Africans in America, health and healing practices were not static sets of beliefs but part of a dynamic struggle to maintain and reconstruct viable institutional approaches to human survival and interpersonal relations under the harsh conditions of European oppression. For Africans, health beliefs and practices, however, were always profoundly related to the issue of how to live. They included physical and spiritual components, remedies for interpersonal problems, and guidelines for living in harmony with nature.[9]

Eurocentric scholarship tends to emphasize the magico-religious components of African and African-American medical traditions. As a consequence, we may form the erroneous conclusion that only magico-religious medical traditions properly belong to African Americans. We may also fallaciously infer that empirical and physical approaches to health care properly belong to so-called White medical traditions.[10] Moreover, distortions and misconceptions about the relationship between magico-religious elements and the physical components of African medical traditions are common. Similarly, there is a tendency to ignore how African medicine has influenced modern professional medical practices and European and Asian medical traditions.[11]

CLASSICAL AFRICAN MEDICINE

African medical traditions have evolved with a tremendous continuity of structure despite extensive diffusion and a changing social context over time. The centerpiece of this continuity of structure is the underlying persistence of a view of reality that links spiritual and physical dimensions and a naturalistic orientation. The roots of the worldview that embodied African medical traditions were focused in ancient African civilizations that grew up in the Nile Valley. Known today by its Greek-derived name, Egypt, this region in ancient times was indigenously called Kemet.

Ancient Kemet produced significant contributions to medical knowledge that were quite advanced. This knowledge had a significant impact on nonindigenous groups who visited the region and attended Kemetic institutions of higher learning and who later invaded and occupied the region. Ancient African medical traditions were spread to Europeans through the Greeks and through the influences of Islamic Africans called Moors.[12] Numerous ancient medical texts were found in Africa, many of which were stolen by European treasure hunters. Examples of these texts were the Heart Papyrus, the Kahun Papyrus, the London Medical Papyrus, the Ebers Papyrus, the Edwin Smith Surgical Papyrus, the Chester Beatty Papyrus, and the Berlin Medical Papyrus. These papyri date between the 3d and the 19th dynasties of the Pharaonic period, or approximately between 3000 B.C.E. (Before the Christian Era) and 1200 B.C.E.[13]

The various medical papyri include both physical (scientific) remedies and magical incantations. Diop noted that "in order for the magical formula to be effective, it had to be supplemented with a drug."[14] The combining of ritualistic (magical) and physical treatments was to become a persistent characteristic of African medical traditions. Another early form of medical knowledge developed and practiced by ancient Africans was dietetics, which regulated the diet to cure varying ailments.[15] The Edwin Smith Surgical Papyrus (2600 B.C.E.) describes 48 cases of bone surgery and external pathology. It also explains methods of repairing fractures that involve the use of casts and splints and of binding wounds with clamps, sutures, and adhesive plaster.[16] The Ebers Papyrus (1500 B.C.E) contains, besides magical formulas, information on intestinal diseases, helminthiasis, ophthalmology, dermatology, gynecology, obstetrics, pregnancy diagnosis, contraception, dentistry, tumors, fractures, burns, the surgical treatment of abscesses, the movement of the heart, the pulse, and diagnostic percussion.[17]

Kemet produced an extraordinarily prominent physician named Imhotep. Imhotep was the vizier, architect, and physician of King Zoser of the Third Dynasty (about 2980 B.C.E.). He is believed by some to have written the Edwin Smith Surgical Papyrus.[18] Kemetic peoples deified Imhotep under the name of Imouthes, and the ancient Greeks identified him with Askelepios, their god of medicine.[19]

Classical African medical traditions were guided by a view of reality that always recognized an interconnection between physical and spiritual realities and emphasized the importance of harmony and balance in nature. This view of reality was expressed in the concept of Ma'at, which roughly means justice, truth, and harmony. It refers to right attitude and right action and to the need to establish the proper relationship between humans and between humans and God, the cosmos, and nature. Thus, Ma'at is the principle of universal order, and health involves harmonizing with that universal order. Therefore, classical African medicine established the foundation of the African concept that disease is disharmony or imbalance that must be restored.[20]

In the classical African worldview, all things are connected. The Kemetic concept of reality envisions a single, self-created godhead with all life pulsating outward as an emanation of this single creative intelligence. Lesser gods and beings are manifestations and incarnations of this one godhead. Humans are forms that exist at the periphery of these incarnations and move back in time through the cycle of death and resurrection to return to the godhead. The cycle of life is like breathing. Creation and emanation are a great exhalation, and the return to the godhead is the inhalation. Spirit and matter are complementary and consist of the same stuff. They appear as dualities but exist within one another. Kemetic gods and goddesses are metaphors for a holistic cosmogony that sees a fundamental unity in opposite qualities found in nature. Life is always coming into being and moving back in time (returning to the source); it is driven by an invisible life force that in Kemetic terms is called the Ka.[21] The classical African view of reality can, and has, taken many forms over time yet persists with stunning continuity within the broad spectrum of African cultures.[22]

TRADITIONAL AFRICAN MEDICINE

Traditional African medicine refers to the diverse forms of health and healing practices that evolved among the literally thousands of ethnic and religious groups that are indigenous to Africans on the continent and to those who have migrated to other regions.[23] The linkages to classical African traditions and the shear size, diversity, breadth, and depth of the therapeutic approaches included in African medical traditions suggest that it is difficult to find a therapeutic tradition that is not represented in the African cultures. Obviously, some therapeutic approaches practiced by one group may not have been practiced by others or been as highly developed. However, even though one cannot classify the therapeutic approaches of each ethnic or religious group, one will find substantial unity, continuity, and consistency in their underlying approaches to medical treatment. African medical practices are fundamentally religious and connected to a common religious cosmology.

Traditional African religions apply to the whole of existence and are not differentiated from a secular world. Religions are communal and not individualistic. Reality consists of God, who is the genesis of all things; lesser deities or spirits who are aspects of the one God; spirits of humans who lived long ago; living human beings and those who have yet to be born; animals and plants; and objects and phenomena that lack biological life. The deceased who are remembered by the community are the living dead. Africans typically view God as all-powerful, all-knowing, and both transcendent and immanent. God is self-created and reachable at any place and time, but there are no physical representations of God. Traditional Africans regularly acknowledge God through songs, prayers, names, myths, stories, religious ceremonies, proverbs, and the like, but they also acknowledge that spirits and the living dead have ongoing interactions in the day-to-day lives of the people.[24]

In concert with classical African medicine, traditional medicine sees disease as personal and collective disharmony. The ill person is out of balance physically, spiritually, and with the community. In one ethnic group, for example, mental illness is conceptualized as a disharmony or disruption of the personality brought about by possession by a spirit, which may be benign or malevolent. Exorcism of the offending spirit to reintegrate the destabilized personality is required, and dance therapy is a common mode of treatment.[25] Kiteme explained, "Traditional doctors seek to create harmony between the body and the mind and with the world surrounding their people."[26] African medicine sees a "causal link between disturbed social relations and disease or misfortune."[27] As a consequence, the underlying stress, which is the precondition for illness, must be removed.

African medical practitioners work with the understanding of how their patients view the world and then apply spiritual and physical remedies. They spend significant time analyzing the health problem and pinpointing the patient's mental state and physical imbalance. All health seeking is not the same, however. Treatment, for example, may extend from self-care to professional physical or spiritual care. Individuals and families may apply their own remedies first. If there is no success, a professional will be consulted who applies physical remedies. If physical remedies are unsuccessful, spiritual causes must be suspected. However, sickness may occur in obvious conjunction with some crisis in social relations, in which case, spiritual causes will be considered initially. The disease may be from natural causes or it may be the result of the ill will and ill action of another or by the intrusion of a wayward spirit. The medical practitioner must discern the proper cause and apply the proper remedy. Moreover, the healer is expected to be able to predict danger and to remove the sources of misfortune or failure. An important concern of the patient is to discover the cause of the affliction. Mbiti noted that even if, for example, the patient is stung by a mosquito and gets malaria, he or she will want to know why.[28]

Traditional African medical practitioners must have the appropriate training and are the people's greatest source of help.[29] An individual may make a personal decision or be called to become a medical practitioner at any time. The call may come through ancestors who appear through dreams or visions. In addition, children may inherit the profession from parents or other family members. Regardless of the method of recruitment, there is an extended period of formal or informal training, usually through some system of apprenticeship. Trainees must learn a wide range of therapeutic and diagnostic techniques, including the medicinal qualities of roots, leaves, barks, grasses, fruits, minerals, insects, bones, various types of smoke used as an inhalant, animal and insect excretions, and other substances. They must learn the causes and prevention of misfortune and suffering and how to detect and combat witchcraft and sorcery. Trainees must learn the proper handling of spirits and the living dead. Public initiations are used in some cases to inform the people of the novice practitioner's qualifications, and some medical practitioners form associations or corporations.[30]

People expect medical practitioners to live by a code of ethics and be trustworthy, morally upright, and willing to serve. Practitioners must not charge exorbitant prices or become rich off their patients. They must use their abilities to help and not harm. Moreover, all medical practitioners do not have the same qualifications, and age and length of practice help to differentiate their abilities.[31]

Traditional African medical practice is further distinguished by specialists, examples of which are mediums and diviners. Mediums are individuals who are able to undergo possession by spirits in order to obtain information. This information may be used to locate a lost object or to discover the cause of a disease. When possessed, mediums can touch or lick hot objects without being harmed and perform other apparently superhuman acts. Sometimes they speak a language unknown to them before becoming possessed. Nevertheless, possession causes the person to express qualities that are not his or her own but those of the spirit. The diviner interprets information from the spirit world. The Yoruba, for example, have a complex system of divining called Ifa. Diviners and mediums also require specialized training, even though some may be born with these gifts.[32] Diverse African cultures may assign the roles of medical specialists differently, but divination and spirit possession are generally crucial components of diagnosis and treatment. Medical practitioners, diviners, and mediums are important mediators between God and humans and symbolize the spiritual view of reality embodied in African cultures.

As the African peoples are becoming able to emerge from the stifling effects of European oppression and domination resulting from chattel slavery and colonialism, traditional African medicine is beginning to adapt and express itself in modern terms. Current research and theorizing indicate that much of traditional African medicine is consistent with modern scientific knowledge. However, more research is needed to fully comprehend the curative dimensions of African medicine in scientific terms and to expand the limitations of scientific philosophy to fully incorporate the holistic and interconnected character of therapy expressed through the progressive elements of traditional African medicine.[33]

SLAVE MEDICINE AND CULTURAL FRAGMENTATION

Chattel slavery and the concomitant disruptions to African institutions splintered and distorted traditional African medical practices. Language, religion, family structure, and the like came under severe attack as European oppression reconfigured the cultural domains of Africans in the New World to serve European economic interests. The suppression of African religions played a key role in deforming and fragmenting African medical traditions since African medicine was profoundly religious. Furthermore, the New World setting forced into close quarters numerous West African ethnic groups originating from Senegambia to Angola. This territorial source of New World slaves extended hundreds of miles inland from the coast.[34] The Wolof, Mandingo, Bambara, Mende, Dahomean (Fon), Vai, Gola, Bassa, Yoruba, Nupe, Bakongo, Luba, and Ovimbundu were only a few of the cultures that Europeans wrested to the New World.[35] Despite their ethnic (especially linguistic and religious) diversity, West Africans shared similar patterns of sacred rituals, similar religious views, and similar approaches to medical treatment. Some elements of West African cultures were destroyed, but diverse African cultural surviv- als combined in new ways to produce New World, African-based cultural forms. Old World ethnic identities merged into new ones, but an African perspective endured.[36]

Slaves often avoided reporting their illnesses to circumvent the painful and ineffective treatments of White doctors. Prior to 1850, mainstream European-American medical practitioners or "regulars" practiced "he- roic" medicine, which employed harsh purgatives, cathartics, emetics, hot steam baths, bleeding, and cupping.[37] Moreover, they used powerful and dangerous (poisonous) drugs, which were largely ineffective.[38] The en- slaved Africans preferred self-treatment, and many Europeans, despite their denigration of African cultures, admitted observing the West Afri- cans utilize numerous effective herbal remedies.[39] Whites routinely ob- served Blacks having greater success treating African diseases like yaws, hard-to-heal wounds, and other ailments.[40] They also noticed that some enslaved Africans had a particularly well-developed knowledge of poisons and the treatment of poisoning. Whites were fearful of this knowledge and tried to suppress African medical practitioners by passing restrictive laws.[41] (The African knowledge of poisons was, no doubt, an extension of the extensive awareness by African medical specialists of the properties of natural substances.)

The African medical legacy in the New World was extensive. Sheridan explains that Africans had practical knowledge of variolation before the spread of this form of immunization to Europe and America.[42] Morais informs us that African midwives carried with them the knowledge of cesarian section.[43] The Africans brought specialists in midwifery, bone set- ting, and rare diseases to the New World.[44] African women and men were equally proficient healers.[45] Their treatments included hot or cold infusions of herbs that were prepared alone or with food, ointments for the skin, massage, poultices for wounds, heat treatments, medicated and therapeutic baths, inhalants, substances that were chewed but not swallowed, minor surgery to drain abscesses, tourniquets for snake bites, splints for fractures, and cauterization of inflamed nerves (in toothaches).[46]

Piersen noted that New World Africans were probably central to the discovery of quinine for the treatment of malaria. He also explained that Africans used more vegetables in their diets than Europeans and advo- cated lemon juice for scurvy at a time when the Europeans did not.[47] Preventive and public health measures among the West Africans included daily baths, wearing loose clothing and washing it daily, burning animal waste and rubbish, the use of fires to protect against insects and chills, variolation, and the use of toilets and latrines. Moreover, the Africans routinely practiced better oral hygiene than the Europeans, using certain roots and herbs to clean and brush their teeth.[48]

The struggle against European oppression and dehumanization deeply involved the struggle to preserve African medical traditions. After all, the battle for the bodies, minds, and spirits of African peoples literally challenged the foundation of traditional medical practices. Even though the West Africans brought better preventive health measures, more diverse vegetable diets, better oral hygiene, better habits of cleanliness, and an array of effective herbal and physical treatments to the New World, chattel slavery eroded these practices over time. Impediments to transmitting traditional knowledge, a new environment that lacked familiarity, limitations placed on the behavior and institutional practices of slaves, and additional factors served to erode and distort African medical traditions. Nevertheless, the enslaved Africans made new adaptations, transmitted traditional medical knowledge informally, learned and practiced "White" medicine, learned about local herbal remedies from Native peoples, and explored and tested their new environments for effective medical remedies.

Numerous enslaved Africans gained prominence and notoriety for their diverse contributions to medical care. Morais informs us that in 1788 in Philadelphia, Benjamin Rush, a noted White physician of the period, spoke highly of James Derham, a slave, who had become so proficient in the practice of medicine that he was manumitted by his former owner. Derham had been sold to several physicians and learned many medical skills through observation. He was self-taught, apprentice-trained, spoke French and Spanish fluently, and became an expert on the relationship of disease to climate.[49] Another slave, David K. McDonough, was educated by his owner at Lafayette College in Pennsylvania. He was graduated third in his class and, with permission, sought medical training. McDonough became an excellent physician in New York City.[50]

There were other examples. Caesar, a slave in South Carolina, developed a cure for rattlesnake bites and was freed by the legislature in 1750 for his accomplishments. He was also awarded an annual stipend of 100 pounds sterling.[51] Countless African-American women like Elsey on a Georgia plantation and Aggy on a Virginia plantation served as elders ("grannies") and midwives and treated the day-to-day health problems of the plantation.[52] In Virginia, around 1729, an elder male slave was freed because he revealed effective treatments for syphilis and other ailments using roots and herbs.[53] Other notable antebellum African-American doctors were James Still of New Jersey, who treated Black and White patients for over 30 years, and John P. Reynolds, who learned from Native Americans and was particularly skillful in herbal medicine. David Ruggles, a "water cure" doctor, also made himself a great reputation.[54]

Goodson further confirms that enslaved African women were valuable healers on the plantation. They routinely were called upon by owners to deliver children (Black and White) and to care for the sick. Slave women, like their male counterparts, used the resources of their environment to treat various medical problems. Among their various herbal remedies were Jerusalem oak (*Chenopodium ambrosiodes*) to expel worms; snake root (*Aristolochia serpentaria*) and boneset (*Eupatorium perfoliatum*) for fevers; cotton (*Gossypium herbaceum*), parts of which were used as an abortifacient; and Mayapple (*Podophyllum peltatum*), a highly toxic herb used as an abortifacient, a strong laxative, and a topical treatment for warts.[55] A prominent White southern physician, Dr. Francis P. Porcher, aided the cause of the Confederacy by extensively exploring the manufacturing and medicinal capabilities of southern flora. His classic work, *Resources of Southern Fields and Forests* (published in 1863), described thousands of plants. Porcher's interest and findings in botanical research were strongly influenced by his observation of the healing practices of slaves, particularly slave women.[56]

The survival and evolution of African medical traditions took several turns in the New World under chattel slavery and European oppression. The enslaved Africans continued to look to the medicinal properties of their physical environment to treat disease. They learned from Native peoples, applied their own knowledge and experimentation, and adopted and utilized Eurocentric medical approaches when necessary, appropriate, and possible. However, the latter techniques were not monolithic. "Irregular" practitioners gained popularity in the 1820s and consisted of Thomsonians, homeopaths, eclectics, hydropaths, and others. These practitioners rejected the harsh and dangerous treatments of "regular," "heroic," or "orthodox" medicine. There was a greater reliance on herbal medicines (Thomsonianism), on therapies that viewed the body as self-healing but in disequilibrium when sick (homeopathy), and on the healing properties of substances like water (hydropaths) or substances that were highly diluted (homeopathy) and presumably did not harm the body. A growing objective was to help the body heal itself.[57]

This naturalistic orientation was a form of deviance to "regular" Eurocentric medicine but normative to Afrocentric medicine. A naturalistic orientation persisted among African-American medical traditions and consisted of the belief that disease was disequilibrium and that nature had a way to restore balance to the body. In addition, irregular medicine represented movement away from orthodox medical power and control and toward empowering the common person to deal with his or her health problems. Oppressed and dispossessed groups, of course, had an affinity for this trend of thought. Between 1830 and 1870, some European Americans began to embrace bathing and personal hygiene, a more healthful diet (for example, consuming whole grains), and exercise as key to health. This health and human potential movement paralleled other reform movements that called for women's rights and for the end of slavery. A leader in this reform effort was Sylvester Graham of Graham cracker fame. Ironically, some European Americans began to embrace health concepts and patterns of living that had existed among Africans and Native peoples but were disrupted or destroyed by European exploitation and oppression. For African Americans, naturalistic traditions would survive in fragmented ways, seek new forms of expression, and become revitalized at various points in historical time. These Afrocentric traditions, however, tended to exist behind the veneer of Eurocentric ones.

The other key component of African medical traditions was their religious and spiritual orientation. African religions provided a basis of organization, preservation, and innovation for African medical traditions. The ritualistic aspects of medical treatment were critical to stimulating belief in the efficacy of the treatment, relieving internal stress, and harmonizing community relations. Disease could be spiritual as well as physical and could be caused by either human or nonhuman agents. Moreover, there was good medicine, which could help and heal, and bad medicine, which could harm. The disorganization of African religions splintered and distorted these medical traditions.

African religions persisted in the cognitive and ritualistic orientations of the Africans in the New World. As West Africans encountered European religions and proselytizing and became more distant in time from direct contact with their homelands, various configurations of religious synthesis and fragmentation came about. Generally speaking, more overt and structured religious survivals occurred among Africans in the Caribbean and Latin America than in North America. The exceptions were Louisiana, particularly New Orleans, and the Sea Islands off the coast of Georgia and South Carolina, where enslaved Africans were relatively isolated from large numbers of Europeans. Catholicism seemed to provide a more supportive context for African cultural survival than Protestantism. Moreover, the importation of Africans into the West Indies, Brazil, and the like was much greater than in North America. The rate of natural increase in the latter was much larger than in the former and resulted in a comparatively lower influx of Africans directly from Africa into North America. Furthermore, in North America, the ratio of Blacks to Whites was much lower, and Blacks experienced less insulation from European efforts to obliterate African religious practices.[58]

African religions acknowledged a single, all-knowing, all-powerful, transcendent, and immanent God, but recognized lesser spirits and deities, which were actively involved in the day-to-day lives of the people. Different ethnic groups called these spirits and deities by dissimilar names. Raboteau noted that the Ashanti knew them as *abosom,* the Ewe-speaking Fon of Dahomey as *vodun,* the Ibo as *alose,* and the Yoruba as *orisha.*[59] The spirits are the forces that govern the affairs of the world. People must maintain proper relationship with them through praise and sacrifice. They build shrines, wear the appropriate colors, eat the correct foods, and observe the required taboos in order to maintain harmony.[60] Chattel slavery caused the integration of diverse deities, spirituals, and rituals, and under Catholicism, African spirits and deities became the Catholic saints. This pattern of religious syncretism was reproduced in multiple locations: *Voodoo* in Haiti, Louisiana, and the Sea Islands; *Shango* in Trinidad-Tobago, Jamaica, and Brazil, and elsewhere in South America; *Curanderismo* in Mexico and the southwestern United States; and *Santeria* in Cuba, Puerto Rico, and among similar settlements of these ethnic groups in the United States.[61] These syncretic, African-based religious traditions in the New World perpetuated a cognitive foundation for medical practices that saw the mind, the body, and the spiritual world as inseparable and the fundamental problem of life as the maintenance of balance and harmony with nature, God, and the spirit world.

The magical and medical aspects of African religious survivals persisted in the New World, but in North America, they became more fragmented and separated from their religious moorings. The suppression of the religious component of Voodoo, for example, heightened the emphasis on magic (control through ritual).[62] Moreover, as the magical aspect predominated, commercialism, through the selling of protective amulets and other related paraphernalia, increased.[63] Furthermore, Eurocentric religious intolerance misrepresented and vilified the syncretic religion of Voodoo; the name itself, according to Hurston, is a mislabeling.[64] In North America, *conjuring* and *hoodoo* were the terms applied to New-World African magic. "Roots" was the term used by southern African Americans to describe healing with herbs, but since magical practitioners also used roots, the three terms, roots, root doctoring, and hoodoo, became synonymous. These practitioners, in slavery and out, adopted the prevailing religious practices and symbolism of the region and utilized the flora, fauna, and other resources of their surrounding environment. All hoodoo doctors and conjurers used herbs, but all root doctors did not practice magic. Hoodoo doctors and conjurers, although practitioners of the healing arts, focused on addressing misfortune and problems in interpersonal relationships. They hexed others; removed hexes; returned lost lovers, husbands, and wives; settled legal disputes; resolved problems of loneliness; solved financial problems; punished tyrants; restored or ended friendships; and the like.[65]

POST-SLAVERY, RURAL, AND URBAN TRENDS

Subsequent to the slave experience, magical (ritualistic) practices to address misfortune and interpersonal problems and the use of an array of herbal remedies and other natural substances for self-care were fairly widespread. However, such approaches could not have exhausted the full range of indigenous African-American health care practices; nonetheless, a restricted and static view of what African Americans did for their health is emphasized in much of the literature. Fundamentally, African Americans used whatever was available to them from their environments to address their health problems. They were overwhelmingly rural and poor, and chattel slavery had been replaced by a new system of exploitation characterized by peonage, intense racial segregation, and radical White supremacy. These conditions further suppressed and impeded the refinement and elevation of indigenous and progressive health care traditions.

To understand the evolution and character of the indigenous African-American medical traditions, we must keep several additional details in mind. There are those beliefs and methods that are practiced by lay persons, and there are those that are practiced by professional and specialized healers. Frequently, this distinction and disparity in knowledge are ignored when it comes to African Americans. Moreover, there is variation in the belief, knowledge, training, ethics, and effectiveness of indigenous healers. Folk, popular, and alternative health care in the African-American community are very much a function of one "racial" group preempting the ability by another to define reality. This relationship impedes the oppressed group's ability to train, regulate, and differentiate, in terms of quality, function, and need, indigenous healing practitioners and practices. This type of situation severely distorts what indigenous healers must do to gain legitimacy, acquire training, and develop a commercially viable practice. What is most important is the persistent cognitive dimension that defines an indigenous African-American approach to health and healing. Moreover, practitioners may express this tradition through individual enterprises, religious institutions, and competing alternative systems of health care that have achieved institutional standing and some degree of societal legitimacy. Orthodox or mainstream medicine may also be a feasible option to the degree that it allows the expression of the extant indigenous tradition. African Americans are attracted to these alternatives based on their congruence with personal health beliefs, practices, and patterns of self-care.

From Puckett's work on folk beliefs we can extract examples of some of the types of remedies used by southern, rural African Americans. These beliefs and practices most likely reflect those that were in existence following the Civil War. Puckett acknowledged his inability to distinguish effective remedies from ineffective ones but nonetheless saw parallels with African traditions and noted the importance of ritual. Several remedies included buzzard grease for stiff joints and a bath in sassafras root (*Sassafras albidium*) tea, red oak bark (*Quercus rubra*) tea, or a tea made from mullein flowers (*Verbascum thapsus*) for backache. A tea made from poke root (*Phytolacca americana*), alum, and salt boiled together was used for a liniment. For chills, one indigenous healer recommended a tea made from willow roots (*Salix* species) and sprigs with nine drops of turpentine and nine drops of camphor, sweetened with sugar. Red or black snakeroot (*Aristolochia serpentaria*) tea was for the chills and fever of malaria, and the roots were to be obtained in the spring when the sap is high. Also for chills and fever, the patient might be bathed in a tea of red oak bark (*Quercus rubra*), eight drops of turpentine, and a handful of salt. For fever, the patient's forehead or entire body might be wrapped in the leaves of the castor oil plant (*Ricinus communis*). For sore throats, patients gargled with salt and pepper (probably red pepper, *Capsicum frutescens*) or with a tea of black pepper (*Piper nigrum*) and vinegar.[66]

Puckett gives other examples. Tea made of hog's hoof (from the pig) may be used for colds; the smoke of burning cotton rags and sugar may be sniffed for catarrh, and goose grease rubbed on the chest is good for respiratory disorders. Treatment for a nail stuck in the foot consists of fat meat and a penny bound to the puncture. A poultice of elderberry leaves (*Sambucus canadensis*) or Jimson weed (*Datura stramonium*) was used to relieve boils. Red sassafras (*Sassafras albidium*) tea was used to "purify the blood" and as a general cure-all. Asafetida (*Ferula asafetida*) was worn in a pouch around the neck to prevent disease.[67]

In the postbellum rural South, some African-American healers and lay persons used magical (ritualistic) approaches in preventive and curative medicine. For example, for chills you cut out as many knots (eyes) from a potato as you have chills and give it to a hog who "will eat the chill" with the potato.[68] The transference of a characteristic symptom or ailment to or from an animal or human was connected to African traditions. However, the magic or ritual was done in concert with other physical therapies. Needless to say, without a strong institutional basis for various healing techniques in the rural South, the number of magical rituals could proliferate among the masses quite rapidly. Moreover, magical remedies became highly associated with resolving interpersonal problems. Hurston gives the example of how to make some one "run crazy." You take three feathers from a live guinea, cut them up real fine, and sprinkle them in the bottom of the victim's shoes. The person will presumably holler like a guinea.[69] Puckett also identifies numerous beliefs among rural southern Blacks that were traceable to the English and practiced by southern Whites.[70]

Systematic forms of traditional magic are based on the concept of sympathetic magic (all things are connected), which is either homeopathic (uses the law of similarity) or contagious (uses the law of contact). Given the law of similarity, when one object is made to represent another, the presumption is that what happens to one will happen to the other. This is the concept that lies behind transference. The law of contact says that things in contact at one point continue to act upon each other at a distance.[71] Hurston gives us the example of how a woman may hold on to a man: take a piece from the seat of his pants and attach a ring. Put a fig leaf in the ring, roll it together, and carry it on you.[72] In this case, both forms of sympathetic magic are used with the use of a personal object for contact and the creation of a metaphor for holding the person in check for similarity.

Studies that reveal the health beliefs of southern African Americans in the first half of the twentieth century confirm the persistence of combining physical and magical approaches to health care. However, other factors and variations must be noted. Some indigenous healers and patients couched their interactions in Christian symbolism more than others. Some practitioners and patients believed in and used amulets; others did not. Some patients believed in conjuring but others did not. Older people believed more strongly in hoodoo and conjuring, while younger people tended to reject these practices. Lay beliefs and practices were distinct from professional practitioners, and patterns of self-treatment were extremely eclectic and diverse. People relied on the resources and substances that were available to them. Midwives and grannies remained a tremendously important class of indigenous specialized healers.[73]

Urbanization, especially as it extended into the latter part of the twentieth century, saw a different configuration of indigenous, African-American health-related beliefs and practices. Even though we can safely say that large numbers of African Americans had heard of conjuring, root doctoring, hoodoo, and the like, most did not utilize these practitioners. Magico-religious practices were stronger in the South and in small towns and rural areas.[74] Webb, for example, reported a documented "voodoo death" of a young Louisiana woman who believed she had been hexed. This woman entered a hospital after complaining of chest pains, fainting, and difficulty in breathing. Shortly before her death, the woman related that she and two other women had been delivered by a midwife who indicated to their mothers that they had been hexed. The midwife told the mothers that the first child would die before her sixteenth birthday; the second, before her twenty-first birthday; and the third, before her twenty-third birthday. The first girl died in a car accident the day before her sixteenth birthday; the second girl died from a stray bullet when she went out to celebrate her twenty-first birthday; and the third girl felt that she would die next. Medical intervention did not help, and despite over 14 days in the hospital, the young woman died the day before her twenty-third birthday.[75]

Southern, rural, and small town migrants, and others carried health-related magico-religious beliefs with them to large cities, which became important but not dominant variants of traditional healing practices. Fundamentalist religious expression in the shape of Holiness and Spiritualist churches absorbed other aspects of traditional therapeutic approaches.

Faith healing through prayer and the laying on of hands, prophets who provided spiritual advice and council and practiced a form of divination, spiritual possession (by the Holy Ghost rather than a deity or spirit), and speaking in tongues were further expressions of an extant health-related tradition that had therapeutic import.[76] Health-related beliefs and practices associated with African-based, syncretic religious traditions and traditional African religions are also revitalized and spread by immigrants (Haitians, Cubans, Puerto Ricans, Bahamians, Jamaicans, West Africans, and so on).

The practice of herbalism continues but is not pervasive. The preservation of the tradition has been individualistic but is to some degree preserved through family tradition. The use of herbal remedies has never disappeared in the African-American community but was probably restimulated by a heightened interest in naturalistic health care techniques associated with the Black consciousness movement of the late 1960s and 1970s.[77]

Presently, indigenous, African-American health-related beliefs and practices are quite diverse but defined by a fairly consistent and structured conceptual foundation. Again, healing is fundamentally religious or spiritual. Humans are spiritual beings living in a spiritual universe, and God is the ultimate healer. There are no accidents. Disease and misfortune are not random but rather have purpose and meaning. They reflect some disharmony in life but carry messages of redemption, which must be understood. The physical and spiritual reality merge, and all things are connected. If life comes from God, it can never be destroyed. Death is only a case of changing one's residence. Thus, for some, the spirit of the dead—usually loved ones and family—can participate in earthly affairs, if necessary, through visions or dreams.

Illnesses can be natural or unnatural. Natural illnesses are the result of human indiscretions, extremes of behavior and wrong action that include inadequate rest, poor nutrition, exposure to severe heat and cold, sin, excessive worry and anxiety, and too many toxins in the body. Some may categorize illnesses attributed to sin as spiritual illnesses, but sin is a type of disharmony with the way in which God intended one to live and is thus part of an imbalance in a natural order.

Unnatural illnesses are health problems or misfortune that are believed to be caused by another person who wishes harm or by a malevolent spirit. Some scholars may refer to unnatural illnesses as occult illnesses. Regardless of how this category is labeled, it includes the forces of disintegration that lie outside a person's control. As a consequence, there must be a class of healers or techniques to control these forces.

The use of magico-religious techniques is closely associated with curing unnatural illnesses. In reality, these techniques consist of the use of ritual as a method of reestablishing harmony. Ritual has the psychological effect of heightening belief, releasing a person from fear, or relieving stress. All are important to promote healing or to provide a person with a new direction and start in life. A given ritual—a sequence of actions that promotes a strong sense of regard, significance, and power—must utilize symbols that are meaningful for the patient or client, and it may be used in conjunction with other physical therapies. In addition, the power of the spoken word and of thought are included in the ability to alter reality, and there is the belief among some that objects can be imbued with the power to protect.

Since health is harmony, significant efforts and techniques are used to reveal imbalances in the body. Nomenclature surrounding the condition of the blood reflects this awareness of signs of imbalance. Concern for the viscosity, purity, temperature, and volume of the blood is common. Other signs are the regularity of elimination; the condition of the nails, skin, eyes, and tongue; and the smell of the hair and body. The rhythms of nature, which include the cycles of the sun, stars, moon, and planets and the changing of the seasons, may also come into play as one attempts to maintain or restore harmony.[78]

Indigenous healers gain legitimacy through the success of their therapies and their ability to express symbols and beliefs that are acceptable to the people they serve. A demonstration of their ability to accurately interpret what the patient is experiencing physically or emotionally is important. Practitioners may claim special powers based on being called to heal by God or being born with the gift of healing. Displaying the appropriate religious values and symbols may come into play in some instances. Successfully making the patient feel better is critical, however. Training is individualistic and idiosyncratic since the institutional basis for training and regulating indigenous health care practitioners is uneven, distorted, and splintered. However, traditional methods and beliefs persist through alternative, naturalistic health care systems.[79]

The current post-urban period has seen the more prominent expression of traditional African-American, health-related beliefs and practices through competing, alternative systems of naturalistic health care. Naturalistic health care systems legally cannot, and ideologically do not, use drugs, surgery, or radiation to treat disease. They include chiropractic, naprapathy, naturopathy, acupuncture, massage, colon therapy, and the like. These therapeutic approaches tend to maintain philosophies of healing that view disease as some type of imbalance in circulation, vital force, neural impulses, toxicity, stress, and nutrition. They attempt to rebalance some aspect of the body or remove impediments to the body's ability to heal itself. Many African Americans are becoming natural health care practitioners as well as users. Moreover, the practice of such health arts as yoga, tai chi, and meditation, and engaging in health-related lifestyle change (for example, becoming a vegetarian) are contemporary expres-

sions of traditional concepts. Many African Americans place these practices in the context of a collective consciousness that calls for the elevation
of the African-American community as a whole.[80]

The effort to reintegrate, reconstruct, and express traditional health beliefs and practices through institutional forms of naturalistic health care
has a powerful relationship to self-care and to cultural revitalization tendencies. The next chapter provides an extended example of how some
African Americans have directed an extant but evolving traditional belief
system into compatible options that can be redefined in culturally relevant
and satisfying ways. We should, however, remember that none of the various indigenous health beliefs and practices discussed here are maintained
and implemented by all African Americans.

NOTES

1. Edward Spicer, ed., *Ethnic Medicine in the Southwest* (Tucson: University
of Arizona Press, 1977), pp. 5–6. The literature on competing health care systems
and practices is extensive. Examples of several extended works are David Sobel,
ed., *Ways of Health: Holistic Approaches to Ancient and Contemporary Medicine*
(New York: Harcourt, Brace, Jovanovich, 1979); Loudell F. Snow, *Walkin' over
Medicine* (Boulder, Colo.: Westview Press, 1993); Doris Y. Wilkinson and Marvin
B. Sussman, eds., *Alternative Health Maintenance and Healing Systems for Families*
(New York: Haworth Press, 1987); Walter Andritzky, ed., *Yearbook of Cross-
Cultural Medicine and Psychotherapy 1992* (Berlin, Germany: International Insti-
tute of Cross-Cultural Therapy Research, 1994).

2. See, for example, Michael Goldstein, Dennis T. Jaffee, Dale Garell, and
Ruth Ellen Berk, "Holistic Doctors: Becoming a Nontraditional Medical Practitioner," *Urban Life* 14 (1985): 317–344; Clovis E. Semmes, "When Medicine Fails:
Making the Decision to Seek Natural Health Care," *National Journal of Sociology*
4 (Fall 1990): 175–198, and "Developing Trust: Patient-Practitioner Encounters in
Natural Health Care," *Journal of Contemporary Ethnography* 19 (January 1991):
450–470; Andritzky, *Yearbook of Cross-Cultural Medicine and Psychotherapy
1992.*

3. Walter I. Wardwell, "Alternative Medicine in the United States," *Social
Science and Medicine* 38 (1994): 1061–1068, argues that, despite its extensive use,
the terminology "alternative medicine" is empirically useless because it is a catch-
all for any medical practice that is not "regular medicine." Wardwell substitutes
his own categories of "ancillary," "limited," "marginal," and "quasi" practitioners,
which he developed in his investigation of osteopathy and chiropractic. However,
other works demonstrate that "alternative medicine" is a useful term, which literally embodies curative methods that are intended to work in place of drugs,
surgery, and radiation. Wardwell's categories are not sufficiently generalizable to
capture the complexity of these healing traditions. Moreover, he ignores the extremely value-laden character of his labeling process. See, for example, C. W.
Aakster, "Concepts in Alternative Medicine," *Social Science and Medicine* 22
(1986): 265–273; Cai Jingfeng, "Toward a Comprehensive Evaluation of Alterna-

tive Medicine," in Walter Andritzky, ed., *Yearbook of Cross-Cultural Medicine and Psychotherapy 1992* (Berlin, Germany: International Institute of Cross-Cultural Therapy Research, 1994), pp. 103–117.

4. See Clovis E. Semmes, "Toward Theory of Popular Health Practices in the Black Community," *Western Journal of Black Studies* 7 (Winter 1983): 206–213, and "The Role of African American Health Beliefs and Practices in Social Movements and Cultural Revitalization," *Minority Voices* 6 (Spring 1990): 45–57.

5. Clovis E. Semmes, *Cultural Hegemony and African American Development* (Westport, Conn.: Praeger, 1992), pp. 1–12.

6. See, for example, Richard B. Sheridan, *Doctors and Slaves: A Medical and Demographic History of Slavery in the British West Indies, 1680–1834* (Cambridge: Cambridge University Press, 1985), pp. 72–76, 81–82, 87, 251; William D. Piersen, *Black Legacy: America's Hidden Heritage* (Amherst: University of Massachusetts Press, 1993), pp. 99–110.

7. The emergence and character of a normative system of White supremacy are discussed by Winthrop Jordan, *White over Black: American Attitudes toward the Negro 1550–1812* (Baltimore, Md.: Penguin Books, 1969); George Fredrickson, *The Black Image in the White Mind: The Debate on Afro-American Character and Destiny 1817–1914* (New York: Harper and Row, 1971); Cheik Anta Diop, *The African Origins of Civilization: Myth or Reality* (Westport, Conn.: Lawrence Hill, 1974), pp. 10–28; Chukwuemeka Onwubu, "The Intellectual Foundations of Racism," in Talmadge Anderson, ed., *Black Studies: Theory, Method, and Cultural Perspective* (Pullman: Washington State University, 1990), pp. 77–88.

8. See Albert J. Raboteau, *Slave Religion: The "Invisible Institution" in the Antebellum South* (Oxford, U.K.: Oxford University Press, 1980), pp. 44–92; J. O. Lambo, "The Impact of Colonialism on African Cultural Heritage with Special Reference to the Practice of Herbalism in Nigeria," in Philip Singer, ed., *Traditional Healing* (New York: Conch Magazine Limited, 1977), pp. 123–135.

9. Ibid; see also John S. Mbiti, *African Religions and Philosophy,* 2d ed. (Oxford, U.K.: Heinemann, 1990), pp. 162–176.

10. Robin Horton, "African Traditional Thought and Western Science," *Africa* 37 (1967): 50–71, provides a very useful discussion of Western misconceptions and shortcomings regarding African traditional thought.

11. See Herbert M. Morais, *The History of the Negro in Medicine* (New York: Publishers Company, 1967); Frederick Newsome, "Black Contributions to the Early History of Western Medicine," *Journal of African Civilizations* 2 (September 1980): 27–39. For a brief introduction to African influences on Asian medical traditions see Kilini Iyi, "African Roots in Asian Martial Arts," in Ivan Van Sertima and Runoko Rashidi, eds., *African Presence in Early Asia* (New Brunswick, N.J.: Transaction Books, 1988), pp. 138–143.

12. Cheik Anta Diop, *Civilization or Barbarism: An Authentic Anthropology* (Brooklyn, N.Y.: Lawrence Hill, 1991); Newsome, "Black Contributions to the Early History of Western Medicine," pp. 27–39; Henry Olela, *From Ancient African to Ancient Greece: An Introduction to the History of Philosophy* (Atlanta, Ga.: Black Heritage Corporation, 1981); Wayne B. Chandler, "The Moor: Light of Europe's Dark Age," in Ivan Van Sertima, ed., *African Presence in Early Europe* (New Brunswick, N.J.: Transaction Publishers, 1985), pp. 144–175; Gamal el

Din Mokhtar, ed., *The UNESCO General History of Africa II: Ancient Civilizations of Africa*, abri. ed. (Berkeley: University of California Press, 1990).

13. Mokhtar, *The UNESCO General History of Africa*, pp. 63–67.

14. Diop, *Civilization or Barbarism*, p. 283.

15. Newsome, "Black Contributions to the Early History of Western Medicine," p. 32.

16. Ibid.; Diop, *Civilization or Barbarism*, p. 284; Mokhtar, *The UNESCO General History of Africa*, pp. 111; Ralph L. Crowder, "Black Physicians and the African Contributions to Medicine," *Western Journal of Black Studies* 4 (Spring 1980): 3–4.

17. Newsome, "Black Contributions to the Early History of Western Medicine," p. 32.

18. Ibid., pp. 29, 32; Richard Allen Williams, ed. *Textbook of Black-Related Diseases* (New York: McGraw-Hill, 1975), pp. ii, iv.

19. Mokhtar, *The UNESCO General History of Africa*, p. 111. One scholar has lamented that despite Imhotep's fame and accomplishments (for example, he knew of the circulation of the blood 4,000 years before Europeans discovered this body function) and his anterior status, Europeans have persisted in proclaiming Hippocrates, a Greek, as the "Father of Medicine." See Crowder, "Black Physicians and the African Contribution to Medicine," p. 4.

20. See Jacob H. Carruthers, "*MAAT: The African Universe.*" Chicago: Center for Inner City Studies, 1979, pp. 11–12; Molefi Kete Asante, *Kemet, Afrocentricity and Knowledge* (Trenton, N.J.: Africa World Press, 1990), pp. 82–84, 89–90; Newsome, "Black Contributions to the Early History of Western Medicine," p. 35; Olela, *From Ancient Africa to Ancient Greece*, p. 81.

21. Karl W. Luckert, *Egyptian Light and Hebrew Fire: Theological and Philosophical Roots of Christendom in Evolutionary Perspective* (Albany: State University of New York Press, 1991); Carruthers, "MAAT: The African Universe," p. 18; Olela, *From Ancient Africa to Ancient Greece*, pp. 93–95, 98.

22. See, for example, Diop, *Civilization or Barbarism*, p. 304; Asante, *Kemet, Afrocentricity and Knowledge*, p. 92.

23. Mbiti notes that in Africa there are about 3,000 ethnic groups. See Mbiti, *African Religions and Philosophy*, p. 1.

24. See Raboteau, *Slave Religion*, pp. 8–14; Robin Horton, "African Traditional Thought and Western Science," pp. 52, 61; Mbiti, *African Religions and Philosophy*, pp. 30–34.

25. Lupenga Mphande and Linda James-Myers, "Traditional African Medicine and the Optimal Theory: Universal Insights for Health and Healing," *Journal of Black Psychology* 19 (February 1993): 30–36, 45–46. Dancing, singing, and music (particularly polyrhythmic drumming) are essential components of the therapeutic process because they permit collective involvement and function as vehicles for spiritual possession and other forms of altering the consciousness that are necessary to reinstate health. These activities also help restore community solidarity and harmony. See Mbiti, *African Religions and Philosophy*, pp. 20, 67, 147–149, 168–169, 239.

26. Kamuti Kiteme, "Doctor Still Makes House Calls: Professor Defends His Father's Traditional African Medical Practices," *Ebony*, May 1973, 116.

27. Horton, "African Traditional Thought and Western Science," p. 54.

28. Mbiti, *African Religions and Philosophy,* pp. 164–166.

29. Ibid., p. 162; Kiteme, "Doctors Still Make House Calls," p. 114.

30. Mbiti, *African Religions and Philosophy,* pp. 162–164; Kiteme, "Doctors Still Make House Calls," pp. 114, 116.

31. Mbiti, *African Religions and Philosophy,* p. 163; Kiteme, "Doctors Still Make House Calls," pp. 116, 118.

32. Mbiti, *African Religions and Philosophy,* pp. 167–176.

33. See A. O. Odejide, M. O. Olatawura, A. O. Sanda, and A. O. Oyeneye, "Traditional Healers and Mental Illness in the City of Ibadan," *Journal of Black Studies* 9 (December 1978): 195–205; Mphande and James-Myers, "Traditional African Medicine and the Optimal Theory: Universal Insights for Health and Living," pp. 25–47; Lambo, "The Impact of Colonialism on African Cultural Heritage with Special Reference to the Practice of Herbalism in Nigeria," pp. 123–135; Horton, "African Traditional Thought and Western Science," pp. 50–71; Kiteme, "Doctors Still Make House Calls," pp. 114–116, 118, 120, 122.

34. Joseph E. Holloway, "The Origins of African-American Culture" in Joseph E. Holloway, ed., *Africanisms in American Culture* (Bloomington: Indiana University Press, 1990), pp. 2–3; Raboteau, *Slave Religion,* p. 7.

35. Holloway, "The Origins of African-American Culture," pp. 11–12.

36. Ibid., p. 16; Sterling Stuckey, *Slave Culture: Nationalist Theory and the Foundations of Black America* (Oxford, U.K.: Oxford University Press, 1987).

37. See John Duffy, *The Healers: A History of American Medicine* (Chicago: University of Illinois Press, 1979), pp. 98–104; Piersen, *Black Legacy,* p. 110.

38. Also see William Dosite Postell, *The Health of Slaves on Southern Plantations* (Gloucester, Mass.: Peter Smith, 1970), pp. 8–11.

39. Kenneth F. Kiple and Virginia Hammelsteib King, *Another Dimension to the Black Diaspora: Diet, Disease, and Racism* (New York: Cambridge University Press, 1981), p. 169; Lawrence W. Levine, *Black Culture and Black Consciousness: Afro-American Folk Thought from Slavery to Freedom* (Oxford, U.K.: Oxford University Press, 1978), pp. 63–64; Todd L. Savitt, *Medicine and Slavery: The Diseases and Health Care of Blacks in Antebellum Virginia* (Chicago: University of Illinois Press, 1978), p. 148; Sheridan, *Doctors and Slaves,* pp. 75, 96; Piersen, *Black Legacy,* p. 102.

40. Sheridan, *Doctors and Slaves,* pp. 81–82, 87; Piersen, *Black Legacy,* pp. 109–111.

41. Savitt, *Medicine and Slavery,* pp. 177–178; Sheridan, *Doctors and Slaves,* p. 72; Piersen, *Black Legacy,* p. 114.

42. Sheridan, *Doctors and Slaves,* p. 251.

43. Morais, *History of the Negro in Medicine,* p. 12.

44. Sheridan, *Doctors and Slaves,* pp. 74–75.

45. Ibid.; Piersen, *Black Legacy,* pp. 108–109.

46. Piersen, *Black Legacy,* pp. 104–105; Sheridan, *Doctors and Slaves,* pp. 74–75.

47. Piersen, *Black Legacy,* p. 111.

48. Ibid., pp. 106, 112–113; Sheridan, *Doctors and Slaves,* pp. 75–76, 251.

49. Morais, *History of the Negro in Medicine,* pp. 8–10.

50. Ibid., p. 13.

51. Ibid., pp. 12–13; Levine, *Black Culture and Black Consciousness,* p. 64.

52. Morais, *The History of the Negro in Medicine,* p. 15; Levine, *Black Culture and Black Consciousness,* p. 64.

53. Morais, *The History of the Negro in Medicine,* p. 12.

54. Ibid., pp. 23–24.

55. Martia Graham Goodson, "Medical-Botanical Contributions of African Slave Women to American Medicine," *Western Journal of Black Studies* 11 (Winter 1987): 198–203. For additional discussion on the properties and uses of these herbs, see Arvilla Payne-Jackson and John Lee, *Folk Wisdom and Mother Wit: John Lee—An African American Herbal Healer* (Westport, Conn.: Greenwood Press, 1993), pp. 58, 72, 118, 198; Eddie L. Boyd, Leslie A. Shimp, and Marvie Jarmon Hackney, *Home Remedies and the Black Elderly: A Reference Manual for Health Care Providers* (Ann Arbor: University of Michigan, Institute of Gerontology and College of Pharmacy, 1984), pp. 10, 14; Claire Kowalchik and William H. Hylton, eds., *Rodale's Illustrated Encyclopedia of Herbs* (Emmaus, Pa.: Rodale Press, 1987), pp. 51, 380–381; Clayton L. Thomas, ed., Taber's *Cyclopedic Medical Dictionary,* 14th ed. (Philadelphia: F. A. Davis Company, 1981), pp. 128, 272, 603.

56. Goodson, "Medical-Botanical Contributions of African Slave Women to American Medicine," pp. 199–202; Duffy, *The Healers: A History of American Medicine,* p. 236.

57. Savitt, *Medicine and Slavery,* pp. 167–169; Morais, *The History of the Negro in Medicine,* pp. 23–24, 215; Duffy, *The Healers: A History of American Medicine,* pp. 109–128; Harris L. Coulter, "Homeopathic Medicine," in David S. Sobel, ed., *Ways of Health: Holistic Approaches to Ancient and Contemporary Medicine* (New York: Harcourt, Brace, Jovanovich, 1979), pp. 289–310.

58. See for example, Jessie Gaston Mulira, "The Case of Voodoo in New Orleans," in Joseph E. Holloway, ed., *Africanisms in American Culture* (Bloomington: Indiana University Press, 1990), pp. 35–36; Raboteau, *Slave Religion,* pp. 87–91; John W. Blassingame, *The Slave Community,* rev. ed. (New York: Oxford University Press, 1979), pp. 65–104.

59. Raboteau, *Slave Religion,* p. 10.

60. Ibid.

61. See Wilbur H. Watson, ed., *Black Folk Medicine: The Therapeutic Significance of Faith and Trust* (New Brunswick, N.J.: Transaction Books, 1984), pp. 3–8; Raboteau, *Slave Religion,* p. 22; Mulira, "The Case of Voodoo in New Orleans," pp. 34–36; Margaret Washington Creel, "Gullah Attitudes toward Life and Death," in Joseph E. Holloway, ed., *Africanisms in American Culture* (Bloomington: Indiana University Press, 1990), p. 72; Migene González-Wippler, *Santeria: African Magic in Latin America* (New York: Original Publications, 1987).

62. Mulira, "The Case of Voodoo in New Orleans," p. 36.

63. Ibid., p. 60.

64. Zora Neale Hurston, "Hoodoo in America," *Journal of American Folk-Lore* 44 (October–December 1931): 317.

65. Ibid., pp. 317–414; also see González-Wippler, *Santeria.*

66. Newbell Niles Puckett, *Folk Beliefs of the Southern Negro* (Chapel Hill: University of North Carolina Press, 1926), pp. 358, 364, 366–368.

67. Ibid., pp. 364, 370, 376, 390–391. For further discussion of the herbs mentioned, see Boyd, Shimp, and Hackney, *Homes Remedies and the Black Elderly;*

Payne-Jackson and Lee, *Folk Wisdom and Mother Wit;* Kowalchik and Hylton, *Rodale's Illustrated Encyclopedia of Herbs.*

68. Puckett, *Folk Beliefs of the Southern Negro,* p. 365.

69. Hurston, "Hoodoo in America," p. 387.

70. Puckett, *Folk Beliefs of the Southern Negro,* pp. 358–392.

71. See John G. Jackson, *Man, God, and Civilization* (New Hyde Park, N.Y.: University Books, 1972), pp. 71–73.

72. Hurston, "Hoodoo in America," p. 384.

73. Charles S. Johnson, *Shadow of the Plantation,* Phoenix ed. (Chicago: University of Chicago Press, 1966), pp. 195–196, 200–201; Hortense Powdermaker, *After Freedom: A Cultural Study in the Deep South* (New York: Russell and Russell, 1968), pp. 286–296; Hylan Lewis, *Blackways of Kent* (New Haven, Conn.: College and University Press, 1964), pp. 76–79; Arthur R. Raper, *Preface to Peasantry: A Tale of Two Black Belt Counties* (New York: Atheneum, 1968), p. 48; Hurston, "Hoodoo in America," pp. 414–416.

74. This is indicated by the places where researchers have located data on magico-religious health practices, the fact that the training of such practitioners has not achieved institutional status, and the fact that these practitioners, in a relative sense, lack visibility. See, for example, Arthur L. Hall and Peter G. Bourne, "Indigenous Therapists in a Southern Black Urban Community," *Archives of General Psychiatry* 28 (January 1973): 137–142; Clarissa Scott, "Health and Healing Practices among Five Ethnic Groups in Miami, Florida," *Public Health Reports* 89 (November–December 1974): 524–532; J. Herman Blake, " 'Doctor Can't Do Me No Good': Social Concomitants of Health Care Attitudes and Practices among Elderly Blacks in Isolated Rural Populations," in Wilbur H. Watson, ed., *Black Folk Medicine: The Therapeutic Significance of Faith and Trust* (New Brunswick, N.J.: Transaction Books, 1984), pp. 33–40; Loudell F. Snow, "Popular Medicine in a Black Neighborhood," in Edward H. Spicer, ed., *Ethnic Medicine in the Southwest* (Tucson: University of Arizona Press, 1977), pp. 19–95.

75. Julie Yvonne Webb, "Louisiana Voodoo and Superstitions Related to Health," *HSMHA Health Reports* 86 (April 1971): 294.

76. Examples are Hans A. Baer, "Prophets and Advisors in Black Spiritual Churches: Therapy, Palliative, or Opiate?" *Culture, Medicine and Psychiatry* 5 (1981): 145–170; Ezra H. Griffith, Thelouiz English, and Violet Mayfield, "Possession, Prayer, and Testimony: Therapeutic Aspects of the Wednesday Night Meeting in a Black Church," *Psychiatry* 43 (May 1980): 120–128; Hall and Bourne, "Indigenous Therapists in a Southern Black Urban Community," pp. 137–142; Snow, *Walkin' over Medicine;* E. Franklin Frazier, *The Negro Church in America* (New York: Schocken Books, 1966), pp. 55–63.

77. See Payne-Jackson and Lee, *Folk Wisdom and Mother Wit;* Semmes, "The Role of African American Health Beliefs and Practices in Social Movements and Cultural Revitalization," pp. 45–57; Eric J. Bailey, *Urban African American Health Care* (Lanham, Md.: University Press of America, 1991), pp. 103, 118; Hall and Bourne, "Indigenous Therapists in a Southern Black Urban Community," p. 138; Snow, *Walkin' over Medicine.*

78. See, for example, Loudell F. Snow, "Folk Medical Beliefs and Their Implications for Care of Patients: A Review Based on Studies among Black Americans," *Annals of Internal Medicine* 81 (1974): 82–96, and *Walkin' over Medicine,*

pp. 73–91, 97–109; Blake, " 'Doctor Can't Do Me No Good,' " pp. 34–37; Semmes, "Toward a Theory of Popular Health Practices in the Black Community," pp. 208–209; Payne-Jackson and Lee, *Folk Wisdom and Mother Wit,* pp. 10, 21–26; Baily, *Urban African American Health Care,* pp. 28–32; Horace Stewart, "Kindling of Hope in the Disadvantaged: A Study of the Afro-American Healer," *Mental Hygiene* 55 (January 1971): 98; Hans A. Baer, "Toward a Systematic Typology of Black Folk Healers," *Phylon* 43 (1982): 327–343.

79. See Semmes, "Developing Trust," and "When Medicine Fails"; Snow, "Popular Medicine in a Black Neighborhood," pp. 78–95.

80. See, Semmes, "Developing Trust," "When Medicine Fails," "Toward A Theory of Popular Health Practices in the Black Community," "The Role of African-American Health Beliefs and Practices in Social Movements and Cultural Revitalization," and "African Americans Seeking Nonmedical Health Care: A Study in Belief Change and Maintenance," *Western Journal of Black Studies* 5 (Winter 1981): 254–263. Eurocentric scholarship on indigenous African-American health practices has virtually ignored these trends among African Americans. Snow, for example, in discussing an African-American healer whom she labels a voodoo practitioner, ignores the fact that much of the healer's practice revolves around her training and certification in Swedish Massage. This healer understands the anxiety of her patients who believe they have been hexed, but she herself has little belief in that likelihood. See Snow, "Popular Medicine in a Black Neighborhood," p. 91; see also Loudell F. Snow, " 'I Was Born Just Exactly with the Gift': An Interview with a Voodoo Practitioner," *Journal of American Folklore* 86 (1973): 311–325. In his work, Baer states, "The greatest paucity of data on Black ethnomedicine occurs for its variants existing among the different religious sects exhibiting a strong nationalist orientation"; he also incorrectly labels the Father Divine Peace Mission as nationalistic and provides no further historical or conceptual grounding. See Baer, "Toward a Systematic Typology of Black Folk Healers," p. 329; Naturalistic health beliefs and practices are very much a part of cultural revitalization and human potential movements in the African-American community and find their roots in traditional health practices. See also Llaila O. Afrika, *African Holistic Health,* 3d ed. (Silver Spring, Md.: Sea Island Information Group, 1983); and Dick Gregory, *Dick Gregory's Natural Diet for Folks Who Eat: Cookin' with Mother Nature* (New York: Harper and Row, 1973).

6

An Extended Look at Alternative African-American Health Care Practices

Naturalistic health care use among African Americans is an important contemporary variant of indigenous and traditional, health-related views and practices. It contains the seeds of an emerging health ethic that challenges the ills of orthodox medicine and seeks to control and advance important health-promoting processes.

The data addressed in this analysis examine the health behavior of African Americans who have made naturalistic health care—alternative health care approaches that do not use drugs, surgery, or radiation as therapeutic options (see Chapter 5)—a central health care choice. The primary data for this study were in-depth, open-ended interviews of African Americans in Chicago who admitted to using chiropractic or the similar but smaller and less well known approach of naprapathy as health care options. These naturalistic systems of health care were not the only such systems of care used by respondents, but they served to identify a community of naturalistic health care users.

My involvement in the African-American community introduced me to natural health care use at a time when there was heightened awareness of this option (the late 1960s and 1970s). I later learned, however, that there was a long tradition and a substantial community of natural health care users among African Americans prior to that time. I used a snowball sampling procedure, but a few of the encounters with users were serendipitous. I formally collected data at several points in time—between 1976 and 1978 and between 1981 and 1984. I interviewed respondents in a number of diverse settings that included their homes, places of employment, the offices of health care practitioners, and various public places. I kept field notes on a variety of observations and experiences. Informally, I collected documents and information on natural health care use for nearly two decades.[1]

The current analysis focuses on the 90 African Americans in my sample and other data pertaining to this community. African Americans ranged from 19 to 79 years of age, and most had some college education and were employed in some white-collar or professional position. I was able to maintain contact with and observe 40 of these African Americans for several years subsequent to my first interview with them. Initially my concern was with why people decided to go to a natural health care practitioner, but, for the current analysis, I reexamined the data in terms of discovering what it means to be a regular user of natural health care.[2] The names of the people that I discuss are fictitious.

REGULAR USE DEFINED

The data suggest that there is a distinctive dimension of regular use as opposed to trial use of natural health care. To become a regular user of natural health care, the health-seeker learned to accept or reject specific natural health care practitioners and options without rejecting natural health care in general. Additionally, regular users learned to prefer natural health care approaches in self-care as well as in formal or professional care. The difference between regular use and trial use is illustrated by the following two cases.

Trial Use

Janice, a 43-year-old university professor, decided to seek the services of a naturopath who was widely known in the African-American community for her fasting regimens and nutritional counseling. She explained: "I started going to [the naturopath] so that she could show me how to lose weight, cleanse my body, and eat properly." However, Janice was displeased with her first visit. She felt the naturopath had not fully revealed the cost of the program to her over the phone.

Janice continued with the therapy because she was "so desperate" to lose weight. For five days, Janice consumed two liquid mixtures and herbs in the form of capsules, which seemed to have a laxative effect. She was permitted to consume fruit and what appeared to be liquid protein, which she was afraid to drink. Janice explained the procedure: "You go back to her on the fifth day, and for the next twenty-one days all you do is drink distilled water, lemon juice, and honey."

When Janice broke the fast (incorrectly, she believes), she became ill. She explained: "When I broke the fast, . . . I had this fantastic urge for a liver-sausage sandwich; . . . it was like I was pregnant and craving liver sausage." Janice never told her naturopath about this incident and never sought medical advice. She never gained faith in naturopathy or sought the help of other natural health care practitioners. Janice regained the twenty-six pounds that she had lost.

Janice's disappointment with naturopathy paralleled her disappointment with traditional methods of weight loss, including the guidance of medical doctors. Through Weight Watchers she had lost weight, but had gained it back. Janice also had gone to several medical doctors. In one instance, the medication that she had received made her ill. Janice asked the physician to explain what the pills were, and she lamented, "He did not do a very good job explaining, . . . so I didn't go back and didn't take the pills."

Janice did not develop trust in any system of health care. She explained: "I don't have a lot of confidence in medical doctors . . . , but I don't have any super confidence in naprapathy, or naturopathy, or whatever, either." However, because orthodox medical care was unattractive to her, Janice continued to look for alternatives.

It's something about [natural health care] that attracts me to it, and I want to believe in it; and it might be 'cause I've lost so much confidence in traditional or commercial medicine. And maybe I'm looking for something, at least unconsciously, looking for something to take its place. On the other hand, I can't embrace it wholeheartedly.

Finally, Janice's ambivalence toward natural health care was reflected in her orientation toward self-care. Even though Janice had tried self-help, natural health care approaches—for example, dietary change—she routinely used over-the-counter drugs for self-care. She revealed:

I have [a] very bad sinus problem, and we keep a lot of aspirins. . . . I use more of anything . . . than anybody. . . . We keep some cough syrup. . . . I have stuff for hemorrhoids. I keep stuff there for my sinus. . . . So we keep a variety of stuff, but most of it is there primarily for me.

According to Janice, these over-the-counter drugs worked sometimes and sometimes not, but she remained committed to their use as opposed to "naturalistic" remedies (herbs, diet, vitamins, meditation, Yoga, massage, and so on).

Regular Use

Sarah, a 31-year-old secretary, had been experiencing pain in her joints and, after pondering the type of treatment that she would need, selected chiropractic. She was not satisfied with her chiropractor because "he didn't really go into a thorough explanation." Sarah returned for a second visit but subsequently constructed her own explanation of her health problem and developed a program of self-treatment. Even though Sarah discontinued her visits to this chiropractor, she indicated that, if required in the future, she would seek another chiropractor. Sarah also maintained her faith in a variety of natural health care options, which included naprapaths, colon therapists, herbalists, and lay natural health care users.

Sarah also used medical care in conjunction with natural health care but preferred the latter. For example, she sought medical advice for intense pain that she had been experiencing and learned that she had fibroid tumors. However, the proposed treatment, a hysterectomy, was unacceptable to her.

Sarah went to several physicians to confirm the diagnosis. Each physician stated that surgery was not indicated at the present time because the tumors were too small. Drugs, they said, could be used to control the pain. Sarah did not want to take drugs because "there is a side effect with each drug."

Through self-study and listening to her physicians, Sarah constructed an explanation for her health problem and a program of naturalistic self-treatment. She explained:

I tried to find out what is happening to [my] body.... [The medical doctor] explained to me that during my menstrual cycle, muscles are contracting,... which is why some women experience menstrual cramps.... When the fibroids are present, there is an even greater amount of constriction because ... it causes a decrease in the circulation; and what you essentially have is a [greater] constriction of muscles in [the] ... pelvic area.... The fibroids are causing an additional amount of constriction. So in my mind, I am thinking ... if I can find something to increase ... circulation, then I should eliminate the pain.

I started looking up herbs. First I started cleaning the blood ... because I felt ... fibroids ... would be something similar to ... kidney stones, gallstones because they must develop from some type of debris in the body.

Sarah developed a self-help regimen. She began to drink herbal teas and to include large amounts of garlic in her diet "to clean [the] blood." Based upon her studies, Sarah concocted a drink of beet, carrot, and spinach juice that she learned was "very beneficial for gynecological problems," and which she consumed at least once a week. Over time, Sarah "noticed a decrease in pain."

Sarah sought the assistance of a friend who also used naturalistic self-care and who utilized natural health care practitioners. This friend held certain pressure points on her body at a time when she was in excruciating pain. This treatment was related to the therapies of acupuncture and acupressure. Sarah found this technique useful to manage her pain.

Sarah also talked to women who had similar problems with fibroid tumors. One woman stated that colonics had helped her. However, Sarah decided to stick with her juice therapy and only resort to colonics if the juice did not work. She also added light exercise to her regimen, which included running in place, jumping rope, and Yoga. Sarah became more conscious of stress-producing situations and worked to reduce the stress in her life. She studied nutrition and became more diligent about making sure that her diet was nutritious. Sarah said that she no longer experienced pain after being on her program for six months.

Sarah was typical of regular natural health care users. She tenaciously held on to her right to define the therapeutic process. Formal health care, whether medical or natural, was an extension of self-care. Sarah routinely communicated with other natural health care users from whom she sought advice and support. She preferred to use medical information rather than medical treatment. Most importantly, in contrast to the prior case, Sarah had a commitment to the concept of natural health care and could reject practitioners within the system without altering her commitment to the system.

Regular natural health care users exhibited several broad characteristics. The first was their relatively deep immersion in a culture of natural health care, which involved embracing various distinctive theories of disease and linking their religious, ethnic/racial, or personal identity to a natural health care ethos. The second characteristic was their relative ability to identify affirming experiences that continually supported their belief in natural health care. This included the ability to neutralize the skepticism of non-believers. The third characteristic was the development of a well-defined and favored role for natural health care relative to medical care. When they viewed it as necessary, regular natural health care users sought medical care (or advice) but preferred natural health care.

CULTURAL IMMERSION

Immersion in a culture of natural health care was an important feature of regular natural health care users. They internalized a distinctive array of theories of disease causation and developed preferences for a range of practitioners and methods of treatment that were acceptable to a natural health care ethos. Natural health care use became entwined in the self-image of users in terms of their religious, ethnic/racial, or personal identities. These processes took place within the context of becoming connected to networks of other regular users of natural health care.

Theories of Disease Causation

Regular natural health care users expressed theories of disease causation that seemed quite diverse. However, a common belief was that, despite the reality of external, disease-causing factors, individuals could and should take responsibility for their own health. As Gus, a 66-year-old, retired laborer and chiropractic patient, explained, "A lot of things happen because of our way of treating the body sometimes—we're not aware of the fact that per chance what we're doing is dangerous to our body." Madeline, a retired school teacher who was close to 70 years of age and who taught Yoga, expressed, "You're your own greatest doctor. And I think one of the main difficulties with our world today is that people don't take their health in their own hands." Harold, a 40-year-old insurance salesman and user of colon therapy, naprapathy, and chiropractic, lamented, "Nobody goes back to the old-fashion[ed] way of everybody is responsible for their own well-being, physically, mentally, and psychologically. That's too much trouble; it takes too much time."

For regular natural health care users, a common linkage between multiple causes of disease was that these causes imbalanced or strained the essential, health-producing functions of the body. For example, toxicity emerged as a prominent imbalancing agent. First, there is an equilibrium state of the body that becomes disrupted by things that we do or things that are done to us. Second, the body must remove toxins daily. When this is not done efficiently and effectively, there is an overload of toxins in the body. As a consequence, the body can break down or become weak and ripe for disease-causing agents to take over.

Although some regular users acknowledged that toxicity can be environmental, they more often saw toxicity as the result of improper personal habits like smoking, drinking, excessive coffee consumption, poor diet (taking in the wrong foods), excessive use of over-the-counter or prescription drugs, and the like. Regular natural health care users believed that these and other substances overtaxed the body's organs of elimination. The wrong foods, which, among other things, lacked nutrients and were full of harmful chemicals, poisoned the body while failing to nourish it.

The colon was of central concern to natural health care users because of its prominent role in elimination and the detoxification of the body. A typical belief was that a colon that became overloaded with toxins created a situation where the body may reabsorb these toxins and produce the conditions for disease. For the regular user of natural health care, foods that aided in elimination and the use of "proper" methods of cleaning the colon were important. Cleansing the blood (for example, through consuming herbal teas) was important because the blood could become toxic as a consequence of poor elimination and fail to function in a way that preserved the health of the body. Regular users identified other organs (e.g., skin, liver, kidneys) that were critical to the therapeutic process because of their role in elimination and in detoxifying the body.

Harold provided a typical illustration of the toxicity and balance explanation of disease. He had "lost a great deal of confidence in conventional . . . medicine and started exposing [himself] to material about natural healing." Harold's illness experiences (for example, a bout with Bell's palsy) convinced him that his abuse of his body was the cause of his poor health. He felt strongly that cleaning out the body through colon irrigation was important. Speaking of colonics, Harold explained, "I use that as a way to . . . clean out the putrid material that accumulates"; "taking a colonic monthly is very good for me."

Harold's concern about toxicity was supported by an underlying belief in a balance theory of disease causation. He explained, "Everything in the body is supposed to work, supposed to be in balance, and whenever it is out of balance, it's something that you have been doing wrong."

Regular users typically expressed the belief that over-the-counter and prescription drugs contributed to overtoxicity and were to be avoided. Linda, a 33-year-old postal worker commented, "I feel like too many pre- scriptions are being written; . . . they are using the chemicals a little too much."

For the regular user of natural health care, there was the prominent belief that one is affected greatly by what one consumes. Food and sub- stances like alcohol, tobacco, and drugs were critical. An intermediary concern for some was the belief in the relationship between consuming the wrong foods, mucous production, and disease. Eating the wrong foods contributed to excess mucous in the body, which in turn created the con- ditions for disease. The retired school teacher explained:

Health is preventative. You don't have to get sick. I mean you cause illness—an excess of mucous in the body causes colds. Otherwise you wouldn't catch a cold. . . . You have a cold if your resistance is low and if you've been eating [fast food], then you have a lot of mucous in the system.

Respondents revealed other important imbalancing agents. Poor circu- lation, poor nutrition, and stress are such factors. Metaphysical agents like disruptive mental processes (negative thoughts and emotions) and a weak- ening of a "life force," or the spiritual energy that permeates the body, are others.

Circulation of the blood is believed to be important to nourish the body nutritionally and to remove toxins from the body. For example, Clark, a 36-year-old substitute teacher in the public school system, expressed his perception of such therapies as chiropractic and naprapathy, which use manipulative techniques, as valuable for improving circulation. He ex- plained, "The manipulation is supposed to help increase the circulation[;] . . . just by the increase of blood flow, it's supposed to help rid your body of viruses and diseases that might be giving you trouble." Linda expressed her belief that "all deficiencies can cause disease—deficiencies in certain nutrients the body needs."

Stress may come in the form of lifestyles that distort the body's structure. Poor posture or habitually carrying heavy objects, as a mail carrier might do, are examples. Jackie, a 42-year-old school teacher, explained that her poor posture caused injury to nerves, which in turn produced pain in her hands, a problem she felt was successfully treated by the manipulative therapy of her naprapath. Penny, a public health nurse in her late 30s, related that a naprapath had treated her with manipulative therapy "to relieve the pressure on the nerves and ligaments in the vaginal and groin area." This, she said, "relieved the tingling and stuff in my legs."

Stress may also be a product of one's mental state. Worry, anxiety, fear, and the like can be the source of stress, which weakens (imbalances) the body. Pamela, a 30-year-old college student and user of several types of natural health care options, explained: "When you talk about health, you're not going to be talking about the physical things; you're talking about your spiritual being, your emotional being. . . . Because . . . negative thoughts will affect your body."

The importance of one's mental state was a prominent health concern for some and was further linked to the connection between the concept of "natural" or "divine" law and one's health. Madeline explained: "[The] most important thing, of course, is the mental attitude—move away from the natural law of loving and giving and being nonresentful—that kind of thing. If you move away from those mental laws, the mind will make the body sicker than anything else."

Hillary, a 30-year-old college student, saw disease as a message from God to bring order back into her life. She explained, "The Creator . . . got me; I been too vain. I said this is my punishment." Balance also means being in harmony with God. Harold explained that health is based on "the different covenants with man and God; it's just a way for you to live closer to what's best for you." For Madeline, a spiritual force "flows through us and sustains us."

Identity

A common feature of regular natural health care use was that the identity of the user became connected to an ethos of natural health care. This identity was religious, ethnic/racial, personal, or some combination of the three. The regular user saw natural health care as an extension of how one should live.

Some regular users connected their health beliefs to traditional religion. Christine, a born-again Christian and naprapath in her late 20s, explained, "The only real healing, I mean healing healing, removing the cause of the disease, is in the spirit[:] . . . the kind of healing that Jesus Christ did."

Religious beliefs also could be intensely personal and nontraditional. Jean, a 28-year-old research analyst for a large corporation, explained: "I do consider myself religious but not in [the traditional] sense. I don't feel the need to talk about my faith. Again, that's intensely a personal thing to me. It's like describing breathing."

Rose, a 34-year-old dance instructor, emphasized the interrelationship between her physical and spiritual well-being:

I think that if a person has a clean blood stream, which this is natural. . . . If a person has a clean bloodstream, they're eating the right kinds of food, and they're getting proper nourishment and so forth, that their mind is clear to think better than what it would be if they were not eating these types of food or keeping the system clean. I think that first you have [to live] natural and then you can become more apt to think clearer or you can become spiritual.

Religion was important to many, but the idea of spirituality rather than religion frequently arose. Spirituality had more to do with how to live and with cultivating a "force" within. Spirituality was very different from organized religion. It reflected the belief that God was behind reality and that there was a way to be in harmony with that reality.

Regular natural health care use, for many African Americans, became connected to efforts to form a more satisfying ethnic/racial identity and, thus, a more satisfying culture. As a group that has experienced a unique kind of oppression in American society, African Americans suffer, not only from chronic economic dislocation and collective powerlessness, but also from the systematic disruption of their identity and culture. Health beliefs and practices, for many, became an important vehicle for changing the effects of this cultural oppression. Slavery, poverty, and discrimination produced poor dietary habits and other negative adaptations that many African Americans felt needed to be changed. Madeline criticized the poor diet of African Americans:

Avoid . . . the heavy red meat—avoid pork. . . . And so why put this extra stress on your own kidneys and liver, the cleansing organs of the body. They not only have to cleanse your own impurities and things we breathe in the air, but now you're making them throw off the poisons of the animal you ingested—this dead corpse you've taken in. And so you're trying to do away with what we call the "soul food diet"—all food [that's] greasy—cooked in pork[:] . . . barbecue and foods like that. High cholesterol . . . is the reason why so many Blacks have high blood pressure, because of the heavy pork diet.

The Black Consciousness movement of the late 1960s and 1970s heightened awareness of the relationship between oppression and health-related behavior and stimulated significant searching and change among many African Americans. Michael, a 45-year-old professional musician, noted the influences of the Black consciousness movement and his use of natural health care options: "The revolution [came] . . . in the '60s, . . . the revolution in eating and everything else. And I started following it."

The infusion of a natural health care ethos in the personal identities of regular users was exemplified best in their dietary habits and health-related lifestyle changes. These phenomena included such activities as food selection and preparation, self-help health care, and preventive health care measures. Regular users altered their lifestyles to improve their health, and they developed a clear role, for example, for shopping at health food stores in conjunction with regular supermarkets. They had a well-defined knowledge of where to purchase such items as vitamins, herbs, bottled water, whole-grain products, fruits and vegetables, and the like.

A typical adjustment in dietary habits was to alter the consumption of red meat and other animal proteins. Pork was particularly an object of scorn for African Americans, partly because of its symbolic significance (association with slavery) and its presumed role as a central contributor to high blood pressure and other health problems that disproportionately affect African Americans. Regular users typically either cut down on their consumption of red meat or eliminated it altogether. Some ate only fish or fowl or adopted various forms of vegetarianism. There were, of course, a range of other dietary changes that included increasing one's consumption of fruits and vegetables, drinking more water, eating whole grains, eliminating processed foods, lowering salt and sugar consumption, and so on. Nevertheless, the quantity and kind of animal protein that should be consumed was at the center of the decision to make a dietary change. Additionally, regular users engaged in activities like fasting, meditation, and exercise as preventive health measures.

Inez, a 35-year-old, civil service employee, described the various dietary changes that she made over a more than ten-year period. The order in which she eliminated certain animal products was typical. Pork was first and beef, second. Fish and fowl were next (with fish typically the last to go). Her response also demonstrated the influence of the Black Consciousness movement. She explained:

One thing is to eliminate pork from my diet. . . . '70 was a time . . . of Black consciousness and those were the things to come up about the pig [pork was considered unhealthy and a symbol of slavery and oppression], and I started looking into it. I'm from the South, and being from the South, I was raised on a lot of pork. . . . [T]he thing would come up . . . that swine ain't good for you. . . . I started to listen. . . .

[After eliminating pork], next was beef. That took [six years].

I started to read more about . . . becoming a vegetarian and giving up [beef] too. . . . So I stopped eating beef, and I would just eat chicken and fish. . . . I just felt better.

Inez went on to explain that she eliminated fowl from her diet three years ago and now consumed only fish as the principal source of nondairy, animal protein. Next, she worked on eliminating refined sugar from her diet. Inez gradually made changes in her diet because, as she emphasized, "I'm not doing it as a fad." Inez fasted periodically and sought colonics about twice a year to remove toxins from her body. She also used naprapathy and chiropractic as preferred health care options.

As a final note, regular natural health care users routinely had contact with other regular users. These users were close personal friends or family members. Sometimes the relationships were formalized within religious or spiritual groups, classes that included the study of health arts like tai chi or Yoga, food-buying cooperatives, prepared childbirth classes, and so on. Linkages to other users and supporting institutions, groups, and organizations helped to fuse the beliefs and identity of the natural health care user into an ethos of natural health care.

AFFIRMING EXPERIENCES

All regular users were able to identify compelling experiences that contributed to their conversion to natural health care use. More importantly, however, they were able to negotiate subsequent illness experiences and consistently find validation for a new way of life that involved using natural health care techniques. Regular users neutralized nonbelievers—particularly, close family members—through affirming experiences.

After Hillary made changes in her diet as a part of her conversion to natural health care, she had to negotiate situations—usually at family and other social gatherings—where she found that the food was inappropriate for herself and her son. She explained, "You have to ... try to fix something to eat before you go or have something at home when you get back." Hillary overcame intense conflict with her husband (when she was married) and with other members of her family as she changed her diet. Hillary did not stop, however, because as far as she was concerned, "I felt that I was given a new lease on life."

Clark initially had a conflict with his live-in girlfriend and future wife when he adopted a naturalistic lifestyle. He explained, "My woman thought I was crazy 'cause I was dealing with all this new stuff." His wife became a believer after their first child was born, but a new struggle occurred with his mother-in-law, who objected to imposing an unfamiliar lifestyle on her grandchild. The struggle to implement the diet and health practices that Clark wanted was protracted, but his initial success in improving his own health and the successes that he saw that others having were simply too persuasive. Clark observed, laughing, "As a matter of fact it seems like a lot of people who used to be real heavy skeptics before are starting to come around and deal with a lot of the same things that we deal with, you know—even my mother-in-law."

Regular users typically identified experiences that validated their continued use of natural health care. Some had been in pain for months or years and had found no relief through orthodox medical care. Others were able to avoid operations that could have negatively altered their lives or were able to eliminate debilitating medications. Flora, for example, a 30-year-old, part-time court reporter, initially went to a naprapath at the urging of a girlfriend and because medical treatment had been unsuccessful. Flora had been experiencing severe pain in her abdomen, and her medical doctor had begun to talk about removing her ovaries. She received relief after one naprapathic treatment. Subsequently, Flora successfully treated a severe rash through the use of naprapathy. Later, a naprapath helped Flora overcome a problem with dry skin by prescribing certain changes in her diet. Thereafter, Flora included colon irrigation and chiropractic as part of her health care options. She successfully negotiated resistance from her husband and children to changes that she made in their diets. Flora also observed that her daughter's friends seemed to be overweight and to have an abundance of colds—problems she attributed to their poor diets.

There were other affirming experiences. Flora observed members of her broader family successfully use natural health care. An aunt, for example, was able to clear up a skin problem that she had had for forty years, while Flora's mother successfully treated a chronic back problem. Flora also had girlfriends who had changed their diets and had successfully used natural health care practitioners. She recounted several experiences of her own and of others that involved medical mistakes, ineffective medical treatment, or dehumanizing encounters with medical care. These events and experiences all served to affirm the validity and usefulness of natural health care and were typical of the experiences of other regular users.

Failed treatment did not mean a rejection of natural health care but rather a renewed search, within the context of natural health care techniques, for a more appropriate cure or method to manage the health problem. In addition, regulars users recognized the limitations of natural health care and developed well-defined roles for natural health care relative to medical care.

DEFINING ROLES

Regular users of natural health care also used orthodox medical care. They preferred natural health care, however, and used orthodox medicine only for health care problems that they perceived as beyond the former's limitations. Similarly, regular users preferred natural health care techniques for self-care. The preference for self-care was of central importance because it was when self-care broke down that formal or professional care of any kind became feasible. Thus, regular users developed well-defined roles for how and when they used any system or technique of health care—medical or natural.

Regular users avoided medical therapies. Drug and radiation therapies, they believed, were potentially toxic and disease causing, and surgery was to be used sparingly. Madeline complained, for example, "I think that if you go to the doctor for something simple, the side effects of most of the medicine given today will proliferate into so many other diseases." Sarah expressed: I don't believe in taking medicine . . . because it doesn't cure—makes it worse anyway, you know, them drugs and stuff." Sarah saw a place for orthodox medical care, however: "Now if it's something that's really serious—you know, say if I got deathly sick, then I would take their drugs. . . . But then as soon as I'm all right, I'm going to put the medicine down."

Other regular natural health care users like Hazel, who was in her late 30s, relied upon herbal remedies as one of her self-treatment options. She explained:

If [my children] get the sniffles, the first thing I do is . . . make a catnip, peppermint, and licorice tea. . . . My son got stung by a bee above his eyebrow . . . so we gave him comfrey tea. It's real good for any type of swelling. . . . I had a little knot that came up on my vagina. . . . So I decided . . . to take these herbs and to bring [them] to a boil and put [them] on like a poultice. . . . all of a sudden [the knot] just started draining. And after it was through draining, it went away and didn't leave a mark or anything.

Regular users of natural health care actively utilized medical care to help define a health problem or to treat a condition that they considered to be beyond the limits of natural health care. Injury, severe infections, cancer, gynecological problems, and obstetrics were examples of health problems that respondents indicated were appropriately addressed by medical care. Nevertheless, there were those regular users who felt that no condition or problem was outside the purview of natural health care. The only issue was finding the right practitioner or therapeutic technique.

SUMMARY AND CONCLUSION

Despite medical hegemony, many people remain committed to competing theories and therapies of health care. Naturalistic health care is one such competitor. Regular users of natural health care distinguish themselves from trial users by their commitment to an ethos of natural health care. Their commitment is not affected by failed treatment or negative therapeutic encounters; instead, they are capable of moving within a natural health care culture to find satisfying and affirming experiences.

The context, processes, and conditions that shaped the commitment to regular use were cultural immersion, affirming experiences, and the ability to define roles for competing systems of health care. Cultural immersion involved the internalization of a naturalistic theory of disease distinguished by the idea that poor health is the result of biological and metaphysical imbalances in the body. Toxicity, nutritional deficiency, lifestyle stress that produces structural imbalances like poor posture, emotional stressors like fear or worry, imbalances in the flow of the body's "life force," or simply being out of harmony with "the way God wants you to live" were examples of the many variations of disease causation that emanated from the concept that a body in balance brings health. The use of the term "natural" implies that there is a way that people are supposed to live, and health is hypothesized as the result of living correctly.

Cultural immersion also involved linking one's religious, ethnic/racial, or personal identity to a natural health care ethos. Regular users saw themselves in terms of a specific way of life that, in their view, was important in defining who they were. This view embodied an ideal that said, "This is the way I should be." Such a view had implications for social change because of its inherent idealistic qualities. Some African Americans, for example, saw natural health care as an extension of their efforts to overcome oppression and elevate their status in American society.

Regular users had moved far beyond the decision to go to a natural health care practitioner. The decision to use natural health care usually involved a compelling set of experiences, but regular users successfully negotiated subsequent health problems and the resistance and skepticism of nonbelievers. They generally reached a stage in their experiences where they favorably could compare themselves to the time before they changed to natural health care, and they could identify others who successfully used natural health care. In addition, regular users could identify the negative experiences of others who failed to take advantage of natural health care.

Finally, the regular user developed clear priorities and preferences with respect to natural health care use. Self-care, using naturalistic techniques, was first. Professional natural health care was preferred over professional medical care. Orthodox medicine remained an important health care option for regular users of natural health care but was confined to a secondary role. Medical care was used by regular users of natural health care to help define a health problem or provide care that they considered beyond the limitations of natural health care. Regular users generally placed limitations on the use of medical care in order to control its iatrogenic properties.

What emerged from the data were people who sought to control their own health. They refused to give absolute control of their bodies to any type of health care professional. The selective use of formal or professional health care was an extension of self-care, and regular users of natural health care were people who were attempting to make decisions about how they should live and what could and should be done to their bodies. The right to control one's body is an increasingly important social issue, and despite the problems that may be inherent in naturalistic health care, it is, at the least, important because it illuminates the strengths and weaknesses of orthodox medicine and provides alternatives to the limitations of medical care and its constraints on human freedom, in the light of growing medical hegemony.

Naturalistic health practices among African Americans embody in new ways earlier traditional African health care approaches. For example, they perpetuate the view that health is a function of interpersonal, spiritual, and ecological equilibrium. Naturalistic health practices tend to revitalize and preserve the African and African-American tradition that health is fundamentally religious and connected to how God wants you to live. They encourage health awareness, a willingness to take responsibility for one's health, self-help efforts, and a community of health activists. Natural health behavior is a dynamic trend that holds potential for developing a progressive health ethic.

Next we will examine the intersection of racism in orthodox medical care and inherent contradictions in medicine's mode of organization.

NOTES

1. See the following three articles by Clovis E. Semmes, "Nonmedical Illness Behavior: A Model of Patients Who Seek Alternatives to Allopathic Medicine," *Journal of Manipulative and Physiological Therapeutics* 13 (October 1990): 427–436; "When Medicine Fails: Making the Decision to Seek Natural Health Care," *National Journal of Sociology* (Fall 1990): 175–198; and "Developing Trust: Patient-Practitioner Encounters in Natural Health Care," *Journal of Contemporary Ethnography* (January 1991): 450–470.

2. Ibid.

7

Racism, the Medical-Industrial Complex, and Post-Industrialism

Today, in race relations, social intercourse is more fluid and liberal than it was in the post–Civil Rights era. Mainstream American society now deems overt expressions of prejudice and discrimination as socially incorrect. However, racial inequity resides in historically based institutional arrangements and becomes more visible when established positions of economic power and political control are threatened. For African Americans, profound inequalities remain in economic development, education, and labor force participation; in access to power, resources, and ownership; and in the capacity to define one's self and society.

With regard to health, African-American scholars have argued, and I agree, "that specific problems faced by the black community prevent them from developing the health practices necessary for a healthy lifestyle."[1] They identify institutional racism (overt and covert exclusion of African Americans from the medical system), economic inequality (poverty and other constraints on the ability to purchase health care), and access barriers (perceptions that discourage use, geographic inaccessibility, maldistribution of resources, and dissatisfaction regarding the doctor-patient interaction) as essential problems.[2] Nevertheless, these issues do not exhaust the methods by which African Americans are prevented from achieving the goal of health.

In this era, institutionalized racism, the organization of medical care, and post-industrialism have intersected to undermine African-American health in new and complicated ways. Racism is embodied in a broad and complex cultural dynamic that erodes institutional processes that contribute to health. Moreover, health is not exclusively or primarily determined by medical care. Medical care is an extension of the medical-industrial complex. It provides enormous benefits to health, but it also contains characteristics that impede that goal. Furthermore, the economic dislocation, overproduction, and radical consumption of post-industrial society worsen extant conditions that challenge African-American health.

What do we mean by health? The World Health Organization defined health as a positive state of mental, physical, and social well-being, and not merely the absence of disease, weakness, or disability.[3] Jones and Rice added another important dimension to this definition. They emphasized that health is also the successful effort "to remain free from physical incapacity while maximizing social capacity."[4] The emphasis on a positive lifestyle and optimum human proficiency is in concert with certain traditional African-American views about health. Some indigenous beliefs link health and the religious view that living a good life (which may be translated as living according to natural laws or the way God wants you to live) means that you will die "easy." This means dying relatively free of pain and illness. Moreover, good health means the continued ability to live independently and to meet your needs. Thus, feeling good physically, emotionally, and spiritually and maintaining the capacity to take care of one's self and responsibilities constitute good health.[5]

RACISM AND THE AFRICAN BODY

White supremacy racism in medical and health care necessarily involves how Europeans have viewed and responded to the African body. Blackness is an emotionally charged and powerful concept in Western European culture and long ago became integrally associated with religious and sexual symbolism. The Western European cultural complex, embodied in the medieval Roman Catholic Church, saw sexual intercourse as sinful. The resulting ambivalence toward sexual intercourse was expressed through tendencies toward sexual aberration, sexism, and racism. For example, the antiwitch craze in Europe was connected with efforts by White males to eliminate White women as healers and with a cultural ambivalence toward coitus. According to Ehrenreich and English, the White, male-dominated Church associated women with sex. All pleasures in sex were condemned because such pleasures could only come from the devil. Healing could come through male priests and doctors, but not through peasant women. Thousands of White women were put to death for the crime of practicing healing after the religious establishment labeled them witches.[6]

In European American culture, White supremacy racism produced tremendous ambivalence toward the African body. To the Europeans, blackness symbolized evil, sin, the unknown, and sexuality. To justify slavery, Europeans frequently argued that black skin was a curse from God.[7] Moreover, according to European ethnocentrism, Africans had defective religions that affirmed their fall from grace and verified that they existed outside the human family. At times Whites released their sexual repression and fears on African peoples through sexual abuse. These attacks continued well after chattel slavery ended. For some Europeans, the African-American body, like coitus, could become desired but at the same time despised, feared, and forbidden. African Americans, for many European Americans, became symbols of sin, sensuality, and sexual desublimation.[8]

European oppression of Africans conjured up other distorted images of sexual fear. The African cultures did not have similar ambivalence about sexual intercourse and did not connect the activity to sin or evil. They and other groups who lived in tropical climates and who felt no shame in exposing their bodies were disturbing to the Europeans. The European justification for chattel slavery stimulated already existing neuroses that resulted in likening Africans to apes. European slavers wanted to exploit the African body and therefore denied that the Africans had mental and human capacities. They fantasized that Black men were beasts with oversized sex organs and an insatiable lust for White women. A resulting Eurocentric culture of domination transformed the fact of the vulnerability of African women to sexual abuse by White males into the view that African-American women were inherently immoral and sexually promiscuous. The myths of the Black man as rapist and sexual brute and the Black woman as whore became juxtaposed to the myths of mental inferiority and inherent cultural degeneracy.[9]

White ambivalence toward the Black body was reflected in its most extreme form through lynching. After chattel slavery, lynching became a major tool to subordinate African Americans and preserve White supremacy. Before 1966, the ideology of White supremacy was openly practiced and sanctioned, particularly in the South. The justification for lynching was to protect White civilization from the threat of African-American domination. Each lynching became a ritualistic expression of a deep-seated fear, hatred, and envy of the Black body.[10]

Arthur Raper's classic study of 21 lynchings carried out in 1930 illustrated this powerful reaction. All but one of the lynchings was of an African American. In several of the lynchings the victims were clearly innocent, while in most cases there was serious doubt that a crime had been committed or uncertainty about who had committed the crime. When James Irwin, an African American, was lynched at Ocilla, Georgia, he was jabbed in his mouth with a sharp pole. The White mob cut his toes and fingers off joint by joint and extracted his teeth with wire pliers. They mutilated the body further before covering it with gasoline and setting it on fire. The mob fired shots into the burning body, and thousands of White men, women, and children came from miles around to observe the event. Although Whites also lynched Whites, lynching became increasingly a racial act directed against African Americans.[11] We should also note that parallel to the racist rationale behind lynching, Whites frequently claimed that, because of their alleged uncontrollable sexual passion, Black women were incapable of being victims of the crime of rape.[12]

White ambivalence toward the Black body and the inferiorization of Black intellect has become normative in European-American culture. Psychiatrist Frances Welsing believes that the fear of genetic annihilation and psychological distress over the inability to produce color—color is a normative state of the majority of the world's population—is a principal stimulus behind this type of behavior. However, regardless of the cause of White supremacy racism, libraries are full of Eurocentric scholarship concerned with the size of Black skulls, genitalia, and mental capacity. Every few years, White scholars, who are usually from prestigious institutions of Eurocentric scholarship, resurrect theories postulating some genetic intellectual defect in African Americans.[13] One must wonder about the source of the cultural sickness that episodically spawns these kinds of questions regarding other human beings. This intellectual racism routinely distorts public policy and the production of meaningful knowledge. One scholar noted, for example, that at the beginning of the twentieth century, a White medical establishment was fixated on the myth that the high rates of syphilis among African Americans were racially based. This medical establishment frequently painted poverty-stricken and oppressed African Americans as inherently and morally degenerate and, thus, the cause of their own problem. It failed to acknowledge the social basis of health problems.[14]

The normative dimensions of White ambivalence toward the Black body is, perhaps, best exemplified by observing its foundations in American popular culture. The American minstrel tradition whereby White men blackened their faces and created stereotypical and distorted images of African Americans was a release for many White Americans into what they projected was the Black persona. This mode of entertainment established the normative model for African-American racial imagery in American popular culture. Noted scholar Nathan Huggins concluded that the lust, passion, and "natural" freedom that allegedly characterized Blacks were the desires of a repressed, White American alter ego. White Americans wanted to become the subjective Black that they thought existed while rendering inferior African Americans as a class.[15] Raper, a White scholar and student of African-American lynchings, observed, "The black-faced characters common in vaudeville, in grade and high school entertainment—sometimes in those of the church—are good drawing cards for white audiences primarily because white people enjoy seeing servile and docile Negroes in ridiculous roles."[16]

Through White-controlled institutions of legitimation and the economic power and conditioned cultural preferences of mainstream White audiences, African Americans remain symbols of sexuality, immorality, and violence. These images help to dehumanize African Americans and shift the blame for socially induced health problems to some inherent defect of personality. Historian David McBride observed one of the many effects on public policy:

The nation's health care system could not break from traditional and modern racialist discourse and institutional health care policy during the AIDS crisis. Thus, the health care and civic community leadership for much of the nation's black population was not significantly incorporated into the national health care establishment's AIDS programs.[17]

Like the tuberculosis and syphilis epidemics of the past, a White-controlled medical establishment and media characterized African Americans (Africans and others of African descent) as originators of these diseases, as a public health nuisance, and as deserving of these conditions because of their alleged hopeless sexual promiscuity and cultural depravity.[18] The historic dimensions of White ambivalence regarding the African body also had implications for the character of medical experimentation.

MEDICAL EXPERIMENTATION

Dr. Aubre L. Maynard was one of three African-American physicians who challenged racial exclusion at Harlem Hospital in 1926. He gained by competitive examination an appointment to the hospital's house staff. Dr. Maynard observed:

The use of the Negro patient for experimentation and the development of surgical procedures and techniques rests on a tradition that began with the advent of chattel slavery in America in 1619. . . . In the mind of the unregenerate racist, who, unfortunately, has always been represented in the profession, the Negro was always next in line beyond the experimental animal. Without option in the peculiar situation, he has contributed to the training of generations of surgeons, his fate subject to the quality of their skill and the integrity of their character. He has sometimes benefitted from their efforts, but he has also occupied the role of victim and expendable guinea pig.[19]

It is ironic that African Americans, through the sacrifice of their bodies, helped to train so many White physicians and to advance a profession that excluded Black physicians from its professional and specialty associations for most of that profession's existence. Of course, all medical students, nurses, and other health care personnel must gain access to the sick, who in effect become teaching material. The aspiring surgeon must perform his or her first operation, and new surgical techniques, medications, and diagnostic procedures must have their trial run on human subjects. Although more social and economic classes are represented today, the poor traditionally have been the preferred objects of experimentation and the first choice for teaching material. However, because of a normative system of White supremacy and their initial status as a captive population, African Americans were especially vulnerable to harsh and unethical treatment, and to outright medical abuse.

For example, in Virginia, African-American slaves were used more than other groups as medical specimens during the eighteenth and nineteenth centuries. Africans were most often subjected to unnecessary surgery so that a young White physician might practice a new technique or, perhaps, gain greater notoriety. White physicians displayed clinical materials (diseased organs) for Blacks when they did not for Whites, and grave robbers were more likely to rob the graves of Blacks (and poor Whites) to sell the cadavers to medical schools.[20]

Experimental procedures were more likely to be done on slaves and, of course, to be done without their consent. The prominent White physician J. Marion Sims of Alabama, whom medical history calls "the father of gynecology," originated the first reliable cure for vesicovaginal fistula, a condition that permits urine from the bladder to escape into the vagina rather than into the urethra. This condition considerably lowered the value of female slaves to their owners since these women could no longer bear children. Sims experimented on seven slave women for four years, working without anesthetic but using heavy doses of opium. Sims finally perfected his technique on Anarcha, an African-American women upon whom he operated 30 times.[21]

Sims felt that White women were unable to bear the pain of operations and that his Black female victims had an inborn ability to withstand pain. The reality was that African-American women had no choice. Slave victims became addicted to the opium that Sims used to deaden their response to the trauma that he inflicted. The opium also stopped bowel activity, which otherwise could endanger his experimental operations. As a consequence, these women could suffer severe constipation for up to five weeks—a horrendous experience. Their addiction and bondage made submission inevitable.[22]

Other experimental procedures were bizarre as well as painful. For example, one White physician poured five gallons of nearly boiling water on the spine of a naked slave as an experimental treatment for typhoid pneumonia.[23] Indicative of the routine dehumanization suffered by African Americans, medical journals openly discussed the conditions of slaves without regard to privacy. The discussions were often disparaging and made light of the slaves' conditions. Moreover, slaves with uncommon ailments could be put on display.[24]

Subsequent to the era of chattel slavery, African Americans continued to have limited access to medical care, and they continued to have little reason to trust White physicians. The ensuing system of White supremacy and rigid segregation that was backed by law, custom, and lynching, however, enforced ignorance and imposed an inflexible obedience to White authority. Particularly in the South, a White medical establishment characterized Blacks as immoral and treated them like lower mammals. As a consequence, conditions became ripe for one of the worst cases of medical abuse in this country's history.

Between 1932 and 1972, a cohort of over 400 African-American men in rural Alabama were denied treatment for syphilis. The Alabama medical establishment and the United States Public Health Service conspired to hide from these men and their families the fact that they had the disease. The idea was to observe the "natural" progression of syphilis in African Americans. These men were deprived of care even after effective treatment became available in the 1940s, yet the medical establishment failed to acknowledge any wrongdoing. One participant, Dr. Sidney Olansky, defended his involvement, stipulated that he had done no harm, and expressed that he thought the men had "earned" the disease.[25]

There have been numerous cases of medical abuse resulting from racism, but despite improved conditions stimulated by the Civil Rights movement, feelings of distrust still persist among many African Americans. After the birth of the movement, White establishment attempts to forcibly sterilize African-American men and women brought fears of genocide; however, more recent concerns revolve around the origins and character of the AIDS crisis.[26]

The source of the virus that causes the acquired immune deficiency syndrome (AIDS) is an explosive issue. Many African Americans believe that the disease comes from a man-made virus that was intended for use against non-White peoples and other undesirables.[27] A White-controlled media and medical establishment continually theorize that the AIDS virus originated in Africa.[28]

This media and medical establishment have routinely ignored plausible theories that link the origins of the AIDS virus to European sources. Strong evidence indicates that, similar to the spread of other infectious diseases that were connected to oppression, poor environmental and social conditions, and rapid social change and geographic mobility, the virus was transmitted to non-White groups via exploitive conditions deriving from colonial and neocolonial relationships. According to physician Samuel Duh, HIV is not a new virus that mutated from a monkey in Africa or Asia. Instead, he reveals that there is greater similarity between the *visna-maedi* agent and HIV. This agent has been known to infect northern European sheep, and there is documented evidence of sexual contact between males and human sheep. Moreover, Duh noted 28 cases of deaths from AIDS-like symptoms between 1902 and 1966 in Europe and the Americas. He believes AIDS, therefore, was endemic to Europe but became epidemic when social conditions changed and accelerated its spread.[29]

The patterns of infection in Africa are linked to patterns of European travel and tourism, to colonial public health policies, and to practices of work that broke up families and precipitated prostitution, that were established by European colonial administrations. In some cases, colonial medical officials began an antiyaws campaign, using heavy metal chemotherapy that suppressed the yaws disease but did not cure it. This policy succeeded in destroying the immunity that many Africans had to syphilis, which had been conferred by contracting the nonvenereal yaws. As a consequence, syphilis and related sexually transmitted diseases spread more rapidly. Poverty prevented their treatment, and the opportunity for AIDS to spread was increased since genital lesions provide an efficient portal of entry for HIV.[30]

Health care for African Americans has too often taken place under a cloud of medical abuse, distorted perceptions, and distrust, but institutionalized racism has also suppressed the supply of African-American physicians, nurses, and other important health care personnel.

RACISM AND AFRICAN-AMERICAN HEALTH CARE PROFESSIONALS

We have already observed that medical care is not sufficient to ensure the health of a community. However, institutionalized structures of inequality have constrained the supply of African-American medical professionals far below the optimum contribution they could make to the health of African Americans. The reservoir of African-American physicians, for example, seems to remain at around 3 percent of the total number of physicians. Blacks, however, constitute 12 percent of the population. Parity would improve access to medical care since African-American physicians are more likely to engage in primary care and practice in areas that are accessible to the Black community.[31]

A common justification for seeking equity in the proportion of African-American physicians is that it would eliminate the tens of thousands of excess deaths experienced by African Americans due to preventable diseases. It is unlikely that physician parity would by itself achieve such reductions, but there most certainly would be some improvement. In addition, we should not lose sight of the fact that the elimination of structured and historic inequality in the proportion of African-American physicians is simply the right thing to do and has other potentially positive implications for African-American development.[32]

One could anticipate profound improvements in health-related social factors for African Americans when the full range of African-American health professionals represented by physicians, nurses, dentists, pharmacists, medical technicians, chiropractors, nutritionists, optometrists, physical therapists, biomedical scientists, holistic health care practitioners, and the like are represented in their professions at least in proportion to the numbers of African Americans in the general population. The services and influence of these individuals, particularly if they advance a progressive health ethic, would be crucial. Formally and informally, they can serve as educators, mentors, and cultural leaders who can contribute to a positive infrastructure of health. They can become guardians against racial abuse in health or medical training, experimentation, and care. They would be an added economic stimulus that could help to strengthen health-related social institutions, and their greater presence in society could help shape public policy and research agendas that would be more beneficial to the African-American community. Moreover, the intellectual and creative potential of the African-American community would be better developed and utilized.

African Americans need African-American health professionals, but we must remember that the accomplishments of these professionals benefit all groups. For example, the work of Dr. William Augustus Hinton contributed greatly to the diagnosis and treatment of syphilis. This disease may have been disproportionately found among impoverished African Americans, but it affected larger numbers of European Americans and others in the United States and around the globe. Dr. Hinton was born in Chicago in 1883 and received a B.S. from Harvard in 1905 and an M.D. with honors in 1912. He developed one of the most sensitive tests for syphilis, and his book, *Syphilis and Its Treatment,* received international acclaim. Hinton became director of the Wasserman Laboratory of the Massachusetts Department of Public Health. He correctly understood syphilis as a socioeconomic and health education problem and not a racial one.[33]

The number of African-American physicians and biomedical scientists who advanced medical care for all people is too great to discuss fully. We are, perhaps, most aware of Daniel Hale Williams, who performed one of the first open-heart surgical procedures in July of 1893. He entered the thoracic cavity of a man who had been stabbed and performed a surgical exploration of the heart. After deciding that the heart muscle needed no suture, he found that the pericardial sac did. Williams provided the necessary suture, and the patient went on to live at least another 20 years.[34] Another pioneering African-American physician, Dr. Charles R. Drew, developed techniques of blood preservation that saved countless American lives in World War II and greatly advanced medical care for all.[35]

There are actually fewer historically Black medical schools today than there were 100 years ago. A White male–controlled medical establishment and White elites who controlled foundation dollars decided on how medical training would be structured. As a consequence, medical schools that trained African-American men and women and White women lost out. White male elites decided what schools would exist by simultaneously creating standards that were financially prohibitive for most schools and directing financial resources to selected schools. Through this procedure elites decided not only what schools would exist but what schools would be dominant.[36]

In the nineteenth century and most of the twentieth century, African Americans were completely excluded from medical education in the South and, to a lesser degree, in the North. The first African American to receive an M.D. was James McGene Smith from the University of Glasgow in 1837; David J. Peck received an M.D. from an American medical school in 1847.[37] To meet the African-American need for medical care, between 1882 and 1903, six medical schools or programs (a seventh existed briefly but had no graduates) were organized in addition to the Howard and Meharry medical schools that were founded in 1868 and 1875 respectively.[38] By 1923 all had closed except for Howard and Meharry. The others could not survive the cost of raising standards for medical education prescribed by the American Medical Association (AMA) and legitimated by the Carnegie Foundation's Flexner Report in 1910.[39] Rosenwald, Rockefeller, and other White philanthropists provided money to Howard and Meharry to expand their facilities and teaching staffs. Howard already had a top rating and fought to keep it, and Meharry needed to work toward such a rating.[40] However, the largest and most successful of the African-American medical schools was Leonard Medical College of Shaw University in Raleigh, North Carolina. Leonard opened in 1882 and closed in 1915 after graduating 448 physicians and 126 pharmacists.[41] Many African-American physicians who later distinguished themselves in their profession and provided medical care equal to the standards of the time were graduated from historically Black medical schools that were forced to close their doors.[42]

African-American physicians had to transcend many barriers because of segregation and racism. They faced blatant exclusion from internships and hospital privileges, and from the beginning of the postbellum period, African-American physicians faced exclusion from full participation in the American Medical Association and its various affiliations. One of the responses by Black physicians was to form the National Medical Association, in Atlanta, Georgia, in 1895, for "men and women of African descent who are legally and honorably engaged in the practice of the cognate professions of Medicine, Surgery, Pharmacy and Dentistry." The association launched the *Journal of the National Medical Association* in 1909, and by 1912 had over 500 members.[43]

Progress has remained slow, and the effects of racial exclusion and the demise of medical schools that trained African Americans have persisted to the present. Between 1938 and 1939, only 22 of 77 medical schools had Black students, and between 1955–1956 and 1961–1962, the numbers were 50 of 82 and 57 of 85, respectively. In 1948, 26 medical schools in the southern and border states would not admit African Americans.[44] De jure racial segregation in medical schools ended in 1966, but the American Medical Association did not welcome African-American physicians until 1968.[45] Between 1920 and 1968 the vast majority of African-American physicians had been educated at Howard or Meharry. Today, other factors such as cost, inadequate preparation, questionable admission practices, and a host of other historical and social factors combine to form race-specific institutional barriers to expanding the supply of African-American physicians. African-American medical needs remain different from European American needs since policy decisions regarding existing or projected surpluses in physicians do not remotely apply to Blacks.[46]

African Americans—primarily women—faced similar race-related trials and tribulations in their struggle to gain access to the profession of nursing. Like medicine, this struggle was complicated by the fact that the professionalization of nursing corresponded with the solidification of racial segregation. Northern nursing schools had racial quotas, and southern ones denied Blacks completely. The White-controlled American Nurses' Association, after reorganizing itself in 1916, instituted a policy of only accepting nurses through their state associations. If state associations barred African Americans, as they did in 16 southern states and the District of Columbia, Blacks could not become members of the national body. Registration for nurses started in 1903, and southern states routinely banned African-American nurses from licensing examinations.[47]

Graduate nurses—as they were called to indicate their formal and specialized training—who were Black suffered routine humiliation and were typically paid lower salaries for the same responsibilities. White graduate nurses were often hostile to Black graduate nurses and subscribed to the norm of White supremacy and Black subordination as they moved to elevate the status of nursing as a profession. Nursing, in its struggle to professionalize, had to overcome a less than respectable image, but African-American graduate nurses had to overcome the added racist stereotype that Black women were inherently immoral. Moreover, to justify paying them lower salaries than Whites, Whites perpetuated the myth that African-American nurses were professionally incompetent. Racial discrimination and the customary use of student nurses as hospital workers meant that few African-American graduate nurses worked as visiting nurses or on hospital staffs. Most performed private-duty work.[48]

Black women and the Black community at large met the challenge to gain full and equal participation in the profession of nursing through great personal sacrifice and collective struggle. Darlene Clark Hine informs us that between 1890 and the 1920s, African Americans created 200 hospitals and nurse-training schools. This activity paralleled the hospital and nursing movement that was taking place in the broader society. The first three nursing schools in America were founded in 1873. There were 15 schools in 1880, and 432 in 1900.

Hospitals only began to gain respectability at the end of the nineteenth century. Previously, mainstream society had viewed them as places for the poor and indigent to seek medical treatment or to die. In 1873 there were 178 hospitals, and in 1909 there were 4,354. By the first decade of the twentieth century, the societal view was that respectable and prosperous people could be treated in hospitals as well. The image that White society had of nursing also had to be made reputable at this time, but for African Americans, nursing had always enjoyed a high level of respect.[49]

Typically, to circumvent racism and gain the opportunity to become nurses, African Americans had to organize professionally and develop their own training institutions. The 1890s brought the founding of 12 nursing schools to train African Americans. Several of the earliest were Spelman College in Atlanta, Georgia (1886), Provident Hospital in Chicago (1891), Dixie Hospital in Hampton, Virginia (1891), Tuskegee Institute in Tuskegee, Alabama (1892), and Freedmen's Hospital in Washington, D.C. (1894).[50] The noted African-American physician Dr. Daniel Hale Williams founded Provident and Freedmen's. Booker T. Washington began the program at Tuskegee under Dr. Halle Tanner Dillon, the first African-American woman physician to pass Alabama's state licensing boards.[51] African-American women took a prominent role in organizing groups and clubs to raise funds to sustain hospitals and training schools.[52] To advance the concerns of the African-American community, 52 Black nurses founded the National Association of Colored Graduate Nurses in August 1908 in New York City. In 1932, Black nurses founded a second national organization, the Chi Eta Phi sorority of registered nurses.[53]

Help came from other sources as well. Again, White philanthropists contributed to selected schools to train Black nurses. Most notable were Julius Rosenwald and John D. Rockefeller and his wife, Laura Spelman Rockefeller. Frances Payne Bolton, a well-to-do niece of one of the co-founders, Oliver Payne (with John D. Rockefeller), of the Standard Oil Company, gave substantial support to the National Association of Colored Graduate Nurses in its campaign to gain professional equality for African-American nurses. Some municipalities established separate medical and nursing facilities for Blacks. These ventures and those of White philanthropists were double-edged; they helped to fill an enormous need, but in some instances they served to maintain racial segregation and subordination. Support was never great enough for African Americans to receive parity in physician, nursing, and hospital care. Frequently, Whites gave Blacks second-rate facilities that they had discarded. Moreover, some White elites were motivated by the need for their Black workers to have medical care or by the belief that they needed protection from a disease-ridden Black community. Therefore, for some, fairness, equity, and concern for the health and well-being of the African-American community were not central interests, if at all.[54]

A few nursing schools in the North admitted and graduated small numbers of African Americans. Mary Eliza Mahoney was the first African-American graduate nurse in the country and was graduated in August 1879 from the New England Hospital for Women and Children in Boston, the first White American institution to introduce a regular course for training nurses. By 1928, the 12 schools that were organized to train African-American nurses had graduated over 80 percent of all Black graduate nurses.[55]

We should note that Spelman had a unique and distinguished place in American nursing education. Sloan informs us that Dr. Sophia B. Jones, the physician who initiated the curriculum and public examinations at the Spelman Nurse Training School, was a Black Canadian who was trained at the University of Michigan medical school. Entrance examinations were higher at Spelman than at many nursing and medical schools, and it was the first school to integrate a high-quality curriculum of anatomy, physiology, and nursing theory and practice with its general studies. It was also one of the first schools of nursing in the South. When Spelman was forced to conform to the practices of other nursing schools, it actually had to lower its standards and abandon its innovative program.[56]

From their earliest beginnings, African-American graduate nurses functioned as primary health providers and not as helpers to physicians. Their active role in the community as health educators and caregivers made them an integral part of an infrastructure of health. In many instances, the Black community regarded nurses more favorably than physicians. In isolated rural communities, African-American nurses might find whole families sick and near death. They took control of the household, administered medicine, cooked, cleaned, and nursed the family back to health. Hospitals that served African Americans learned that nurses who performed important outreach activities were equal to physicians in their importance to Black health.[57]

Like medical doctors, the struggle to gain admission and acceptance into national associations and into all phases of the nursing profession was protracted and frustrating. For example, gross discrimination by the Red Cross and exclusion from the war effort (World War I) was especially daunting. Thus, a particularly satisfying victory was to gain acceptance to the Army Nurse Corps without regard to race on January 20, 1945. A few days later, the Navy Nurse Corps opened itself to African-American nurses. In these cases, activism, a shortage of nurses, and World War II helped to speed desegregation.[58]

Finally, the American Nurses' Association (ANA) opened its doors to African-American nurses by permitting individual membership in 1948. In 1950 the National Association of Colored Graduate Nurses declared their dissolution after becoming integrated into the ANA. Two leading lights in the struggle for professional equality were nurses Estelle Massey Riddle and Mabel Keaton Staupers; Ruth Logan Roberts was an important lay leader in the struggle. Black nurses remained principally in private duty or worked in the higher-status position of public health nurse. African-American nurses did not enter hospital staff duty in any significant numbers until the 1960s, and the change at White hospitals was a response to changes in the civil rights laws. New, continuing, and virulent forms of race-specific inequality stimulated African-American nurses to respond by founding the National Black Nurses' Association in 1971.[59] Through her careful analysis of the struggle by African-American nurses to gain professional acceptance and equality, Hine observed, "Separate institutions and organizations founded by and under the control of black people remain . . . important weapons against racism."[60]

The struggle to train African-American nurses and physicians and to gain professional acceptance and equality had its advocates, supporters, heroines, and heroes; but the struggle is not over. Like physicians, race-specific social factors prohibit achieving adequate numbers of African-American nurses.[61] Furthermore, training institutions and hospitals that service the medical care needs of African-American communities have declined drastically. They shrank from 200 in 1900 to 12 in 1992; 57 were lost between 1961 and 1988. African-American hospitals have traditionally treated the poor. This fact, and rapidly increasing health care costs, have left these hospitals unable to modernize. They cannot expand or acquire the costly technologies that are necessary to attract doctors and their patients.[62]

What African Americans have found is that without sufficient capital, so-called integration can be a one-way path to oblivion. Black businesses are likely to be undercapitalized and cannot compete with well-established, highly financed, White-owned institutions. These economic inequities have already been entrenched by centuries of oppression and underdevelopment. Moreover, African Americans know all too well that individual and institutional racism continue to exist in the marketplace. White-owned institutions also may succumb to changing market forces, but when they do, there are many more to take their place. The same is not true for African Americans.

Thus, what applies to African-American business development in general applies to the survival of Black hospitals. The elimination of de jure segregation opened African-American markets more efficiently to White businesses, but it did not provide a vehicle for Black businesses to gain equal access to non-Black markets. Furthermore, desegregation did little to enhance the capability of Black businesses to compete equally for the consumer dollars of an expanding Black middle class. Because of these structural deformities, access to medical care and the distribution of related resources become even more subject to the whim of White-owned and controlled hospitals and their specific medical and market agendas.

These problems are not individualistic but institutional and are exacerbated by market forces inherent in the organization of medical care and the character of maturing capitalism. They both intersect with systemic processes that erode the infrastructure of African-American health. Unfortunately, modern medicine has not evolved and does not proceed based on the singular goal of achieving health. Moreover, African Americans were, and are, impeded from shaping the professional and elite structures of the organization of medicine, just as they have been historically impeded from gaining a foothold at the level of ownership and control of any significant sphere of economic activity. There is no substantial capital-owning class among African Americans that can compare with ruling White elites. There are no Black philanthropic organizations that can significantly alter public policy through their patterns of giving.

Historically, African-American communities are creations of economic forces that have served the interests of White elites. The end of legal segregation was not the result of moral enlightenment; rather it was a case of a social form becoming counterproductive to the economic objectives of ruling enclaves. Thus, the fundamental problem for African Americans now is the same as it was for Booker T. Washington and others of his time. In a relationship of profound dependency, how do you leverage support to gain some of what you need from ruling elites until you can gain the independence and resources necessary to fully obtain, implement, and sustain all you need? Of course, along the way, ruling enclaves may engage in co-optation if the goals of subordinates do not coincide with their own. Moreover, they act, not only based on their economic interests, but also on their ideological and cultural interests. The goal of African-American health is perennially subject to such obstacles.

THE MEDICAL-INDUSTRIAL COMPLEX AND POST-INDUSTRIALISM

Industrialism is the formation of large-scale industries for the mass and cheap production of goods. It is characterized by urban factories and a growing and sizable workforce predominantly engaged in manufacturing. The historical era of industrialism is one of dynamic growth, despite periodic economic downturns. Immigration and migration to the cities are prominent as people seek employment opportunities created by the increased demand for industrial labor. Urban population growth and growth in the quantity and diversity of goods produced are characteristic. However, what is most distinctive about this period is that the revolution in the production of goods parallels a highly untapped market for these goods.

One critical reason for this type of surplus market condition is that there is a new shift from one mode of life to another. The change from an emphasis on rural to urban life and from agricultural to industrial production massively expands wage earners and, for the first time, spawns a consumer culture. For the most part, the wants and needs of society are no longer met by individual action or familial and small-scale institutional organization, but by the massive collective action of industrial production. There emerges a tendency toward greater and greater commodification, since that which people formerly produced or did for themselves (or did without) can be obtained in the marketplace. Thus, there is a revolution in the quantity of things that can be bought and sold.

It is important to note that in this racially stratified country, European Americans did not permit African Americans to benefit from the economic rewards of industrialism. At the time that European Americans dominated American industrial cities, White elites kept African Americans as an exploited class of agricultural workers and White society maintained a general system of overt racial subordination. African Americans were blocked from equal participation as industrial workers and owners and in related economic activity that offered high salaries or opportunities for capital accumulation. Whenever African Americans did manage to compete effectively with Whites for economic resources, they were simply removed from competition through restrictions on licensure, impediments to adequate capital, outright violence and intimidation, and the like. We cannot review this history here, but suffice it to say, for African Americans, economic dislocation was characteristic of industrialism from its inception. This economic dislocation paralleled an extant tendency to disrupt among Africans cultural formations that encouraged political and economic cohesion that could advance collective empowerment. For African Americans, the creation of underdevelopment and a new relationship of dependency were the historic results of American industrialism.[63]

Post-industrialism represents both a continuation of industrialism and a break with many of its dominant trends. Post-industrial society is still dominated by mass-produced goods made possible by revolutions in science and technology. Rapid increases in the numbers of technocrats, in the division of physical and mental labor, and in specialization in the professions characterize the maturing of industrialism and continue into the post-industrial era. The computerized, information-oriented nature of post-industrial society stands out as a defining feature. Another is the decrease in the size of the manufacturing sector relative to an increase in the size of the service sector of the economy. Technological innovation and the search for profit contribute to more efficient productive forces that need fewer bodies to produce more and more goods. Moreover, where workers are needed, the goal of maximizing profit by reducing labor cost precipitates a domestic and global search for cheaper labor, which erodes an already declining industrial workforce.[64] Because the American racial dynamic made African Americans latecomers and marginal to industrial ownership and production, they are disproportionately and negatively affected by post-industrial stagnation and urban blight.

Several features of post-industrialism that are important to this aspect of our analysis are increasing commodification, shrinking markets, and surplus production. Commodification—the process of creating things to be bought and sold—is accelerated during industrialism but becomes radicalized in the post-industrial era. Shrinking markets reflect inherent limitations on consumption as increasing numbers of goods and services are produced and scarcity is replaced by overproduction and surplus.

The profit and ideological demands of the economy require the stimulation of radical consumption in the face of overproduction and shrinking markets. The need for radical consumption contributes to the requirement to produce new social needs and wants that can be bought and sold and the need to persuade or coerce people to purchase a product or service rather than supply it themselves. To not consume becomes a form of deviance, and life increasingly becomes defined by what you buy and not what you do. Medical care follows this trend.

Medicalization is the radical and pervasive expansion of medical markets. It is the invasion of medical care into increasingly greater aspects of life from birth to death. Medicalization is the response of the medical-industrial complex to the post-industrial problems of overproduction and limited markets and the goal of profit. Furthermore, relative to most other sectors of the economy, the medical-industrial complex is in a more powerful position to control supply and demand.[65] It can greatly determine how much of its products consumers consume. Theoretically, rising costs appear to be the only factor that can constrain medicalization since the structure of third-party payers (insurance companies, the federal government, and the like), which contributes to greater utilization of the medical system, cannot continue to support its excesses. However, despite much debate and concern, medical costs have defied control and continue to rise at abnormally high rates when compared to other sectors of the economy.[66]

Medicalization carries other counterproductive yet self-serving results. One such outcome is the epidemic of iatrogenic diseases. Iatrogenesis is the proliferation of medically produced ailments and deaths and, borrowing from social critic Ivan Illich, consists of three types: clinical, social, and cultural.[67] Clinical iatrogenesis occurs when hospitals and physicians are the sickening agents and their intervention produces additional pain, dysfunction, disability, anxiety, and even death. The side effects of drug therapy, unnecessary surgery and other unnecessary tests and treatments; injury and death from invasive diagnostic procedures; mistakes in testing, diagnosis, and treatment; and the like are examples.[68]

Social iatrogenesis occurs when health is undermined by the social organization of medical care. Here, the radical tendencies of the medical-industrial complex to control and expand medical markets independently of the goal of health are an example. Disease is characteristically socially constructed, but medical monopolies continually expand the boundaries of morbidity and impose their considerable power of social control to seduce and coerce the citizenry to consume their products.[69]

Cultural iatrogenesis is the process of transforming people into consumers by destroying their ability to deal with pain, sickness, and death. It destroys the capability for self-care. The tendency is to make people lose their ability to generate a countervailing struggle against counterproductive medical expansion. In turn, pain, sickness, and death simply become new markets for increasing amounts of drugs, surgery, and hospital and medical services. Illich is correct when he observed that through cultural iatrogenesis, people are trained for consumption rather than action.[70]

Cultural iatrogenesis is particularly troublesome for the health problems of African Americans, as it is a form of socially induced dependence. African Americans, who also are faced with historic and systemic attacks on their infrastructure of health, are stripped even more of their cultural capabilities to address post-industrial consumer manipulation. The problem of systemic cultural negation and manipulation (cultural hegemony) that is characteristic of the structure of racial inequality experienced by African Americans is another type of socially induced dependency. Thus, the intersection of cultural hegemony with post-industrial medicalization creates a highly formidable challenge to the goal of African-American health. The result is a more heightened destabilization of the ability of African Americans to address the more fundamental social and cultural bases of health.

In the next chapter we will look at the problem of socially induced dependency and radical consumer manipulation in the light of current and major threats to African-American health.

NOTES

1. Woodrow Jones and Mitchell F. Rice, eds., *Health Care Issues in Black America: Policies, Problems, and Prospects* (Westport, Conn.: Greenwood Press, 1987), p. 5.

2. Ibid., pp. 5–9; see also Woodrow Jones, Jr., and Antonio A. Rene, "Barriers to Health Services Utilization and African Americans," in Ivor Lensworth Livingston, ed., *Handbook of Black American Health: The Mosaic of Conditions, Issues, Policies, and Prospects* (Westport, Conn.: Greenwood Press, 1994), pp. 378–386.

3. Jones and Rice, *Health Care Issues in Black America*, p. 4.

4. Ibid.

5. See J. Herman Blake, " 'Doctor Can't Do Me No Good': Social Concomitants of Health Care Attitudes and Practices among Elderly Blacks in Isolated Rural Populations," in Wilbur H. Watson, ed., *Black Folk Medicine: The Therapeutic Significance of Faith and Trust* (New Brunswick, N.J.: Transaction Books, 1984), p. 38.

6. Barbara Ehrenreich and Deirdre English, *Witches, Midwives, and Nurses: A History of Women Healers* (New York: Feminist Press, 1973), pp. 2–13.

7. Roger Bastide, "Color, Racism, and Christianity," in John Hope Franklin, ed., *Color and Race* (Boston: Beacon Press, 1969), p. 36.

8. See, for example, George Fredrickson, *The Black Image in the White Mind: The Debate on Afro-American Character and Destiny 1817–1914* (New York: Harper and Row, 1971); Winthrop Jordan, *White over Black: American Attitudes Toward the Negro 1550–1812* (Baltimore, Md.: Penguin Books, 1969), pp. 3–98; Calvin C. Hernton, *Sex and Racism in America* (New York: Grove Press, 1966), pp. 11–54, 89–120; Franz Fanon, *Black Skin, White Mask* (New York: Grove Press, 1967), pp. 42, 141–209; Frances C. Welsing, *The Isis Papers: The Keys to the Colors* (Chicago: Third World Press, 1991), pp. 1–51.

9. Ibid.

10. Bertram Doyle, *The Etiquette of Race Relations in the South: A Study in Social Control* (New York: Schocken Books, 1971) provides a classic description of overt and unrestrained White supremacy in the South.

11. Arthur R. Raper, *The Tragedy of Lynching* (New York: Dover Publications, 1970), pp. 1–7, 12–13; see also, Ralph Ginzburg, *100 Years of Lynchings* (Baltimore, Md.: Black Classic Press, 1988).

12. Mary Frances Berry and John W. Blassingame, *Long Memory: The Black Experience in America* (New York: Oxford University Press, 1982), pp. 115–116.

13. See Robert S. Boyd, "Coloring Intelligence," *Detroit Free Press,* October 23, 1994, pp. 1F, 4F; Ellen K. Coughlin "Class, IQ, and Heredity," *Chronicle of Higher Education,* October 23, 1994, pp. A12, A20. These articles discuss the latest contribution to Eurocentric racialist thought to link intelligence with race: Richard J. Hernstein and Charles Murray, *The Bell Curve: Intelligence and Class Structure in American Life* (New York: Free Press, 1994).

14. David McBride, *From TB to AIDS: Epidemics among Urban Blacks since 1900* (Albany: State University of New Press, 1991), pp. 10, 15–17, 19–22.

15. Nathan Huggins, *Harlem Renaissance* (New York: Oxford University Press, 1971), pp. 253–254.

16. Raper, *The Tragedy of Lynching,* p. 49.

17. McBride, *From TB to AIDS,* p. 159.

18. Mainstream news publications remain fixated on AIDS as an African disease. See, for example, Geoffrey Cowley, "The Future of AIDS," *Newsweek,* March 22, 1993, pp. 47–52. Samuel V. Duh, *Blacks and Aids* (Newbury Park, Calif.: Sage, 1991), pp. 60–66, 69–70, provides a more balanced view and also presents a very plausible and scientifically supportable theory on the European origins of AIDS and on the social basis by which it became a global epidemic.

19. Aubre L. Maynard, *Surgeons to the Poor: The Harlem Hospital Story* (New York: Appleton-Century-Crofts, 1978), p. 3.

20. Todd L. Savitt, *Medicine and Slavery: The Diseases and Health Care of Blacks in Antebellum Virginia* (Chicago: University of Illinois Press, 1978), pp. 281–289.

21. See Robert S. Mendelsohn, *Male Practice: How Doctors Manipulate Women* (Chicago: Contemporary Books, 1982), pp. 33–34; Savitt, *Medicine and Slavery,* p. 297; Diana Scully, *Men Who Control Women's Health: The Miseducation of Obstetrician Gynecologists* (Boston: Houghton Mifflin, 1980), pp. 41–42.

22. Scully, *Men Who Control Women's Health*, p. 43.

23. Savitt, *Medicine and Slavery*, p. 299.

24. Ibid., pp. 301, 305–307.

25. See James H. Jones, *Bad Blood: The Tuskegee Syphilis Experiment—A Tragedy of Race and Medicine* (New York: Free Press, 1981); and John H. Stanfield, "Venereal Disease Control Demonstrations among Rural Blacks in the American South," *Western Journal of Black Studies* 5 (Winter 1981): 246–253; Olansky is discussed in Tom Junod, "Deadly Medicine," *Gentleman's Quarterly*, June 1993, p. 170.

26. See Robert G. Weisbord, *Genocide? Birth Control and the Black American* (Westport, Conn.: Greenwood Press, 1975), pp. 31–34, 137–138, 141–155, 158–174; Tom Junod, "Deadly Medicine," pp. 164–171, 231–234; Harriet Washington, "Human Guinea Pigs," *Emerge*, October 1994, pp. 24–35.

27. See Welsing, *The Isis Papers*, pp. 291–301.

28. For example, see Geoffrey Cowley, "The Future of AIDS," *Newsweek*, March 22, 1993, pp. 47–52.

29. See Duh, *Blacks and Aids*, pp. 60–66, 69–70; McBride, *From TB to AIDS*, pp. 10, 15–19, 23, 159–171.

30. Ibid.

31. See, for example, Moses K. Woode and Kathleen Bodisch Lynch, "Effective Intervention Strategies for Producing Black Health Care Providers," in Ronald L. Braithwaite and Sandra E. Taylor, eds., *Health Issues in the Black Community* (San Francisco: Jossey-Bass, 1992), p. 281; Ruth S. Hanft and Catherine C. White, "Constraining the Supply of Physicians: Effects on Black Physicians," in David P. Willis, ed., *Health Policies and Black Americans* (New Brunswick, N.J.: Transaction Publishers, 1989); Gary King, "The Supply and Distribution of Black Physicians in the United States: 1900–1970," *Western Journal of Black Studies* 4 (Spring 1980): 21; and John Obioma Ukawilulu and Ivor Lensworth Livingston, "Black Health Care Providers and Related Professionals: Issues of Underrepresentation and Change," in Ivor Lensworth Livingston, ed., *Handbook of Black American Health: The Mosaic of Conditions, Issues, Policies, and Prospects* (Westport, Conn.: Greenwood Press, 1994), pp. 344–360.

32. Ukawilulu, "Black Health Care Providers and Related Professionals," pp. 344–360.

33. Herbert M. Morais, *The History of the Negro in Medicine* (New York: Publishers Company, 1967), pp. 103–104.

34. Ibid., pp. 74–75.

35. Ibid., p. 108.

36. See Paul Starr, *The Social Transformation of American Medicine: The Rise of a Sovereign Profession and the Making of a Vast Industry* (New York: Basic Books, 1982), pp. 116–124.

37. King, "The Supply and Distribution of Black Physicians in the United States," p. 22.

38. Ibid., p. 22; Ralph L. Crowder, "Black Physicians and the African Contribution to Medicine," *Western Journal of Black Studies* 4 (Spring 1980): 12–13.

39. The American Medical Association (AMA) secured the support of the Carnegie Foundation for the Advancement of Teaching to carry out reforms in medical education that it had already begun. Abraham Flexner was given the task by

the foundation to assess the country's medical schools and make recommendations regarding their status. The number of medical schools had already begun to decline, however, before the Flexner Report was published in 1910. Higher costs to students and institutions to meet new standards drove the less financially viable schools out of existence. The new standards had to be observed because otherwise, the diplomas would not be recognized by the state licensing boards. See Starr, *The Social Transformation of American Medicine,* pp. 117–118.

40. Morais, *The History of the Negro in Medicine,* p. 92.

41. King, "The Supply and Distribution of Black Physicians in the United States," p. 22.

42. See Morais, *The History of the Negro in Medicine,* pp. 60–66; Starr, *The Social Transformation of American Medicine,* pp. 124–125.

43. Morais, *The History of the Negro in Medicine,* pp. 68–69.

44. Max Seham, *Blacks and American Medical Care* (Minneapolis: University of Minnesota Press, 1973), p. 45.

45. Ibid., p. 60; Hanft and White, "Constraining the Supply of Physicians," pp. 249, 265.

46. Ibid., pp. 249–269. Dr. Lonnie Bristow, in 1994, was elected as the first African American to serve as AMA president. He was also the AMA's first Black trustee and board chairman. It remains to be seen whether his presence will make the medical establishment more responsive to the health care needs of African Americans. See Joyce Jones, "Speechmaker or Catalyst for Change? Bristow Hopes to Help Preserve Doctor/Patient Relationships," *Black Enterprise* 25 (October 1994): 18.

47. Darlene Clark Hine, *Black Women in White: Racial Conflict and Cooperation in the Nursing Profession 1890–1950* (Bloomington: Indiana University Press, 1989), pp. xix, 89–98; Patricia Sloan, "Early Black Nursing Schools and Responses of Black Nurses to Their Educational Programs," *Western Journal of Black Studies* 9 (Fall 1985): 163.

48. Hine, *Black Women in White,* pp. 49–50, 98, 136; Ehrenreich and English, *Witches, Midwives and Nurses,* p. 33.

49. Hine, *Black Women in White,* pp. xv–xvii, 3–6.

50. Sloan, "Early Black Nursing Schools and Responses of Black Nurses to their Educational Programs," p. 158; Morais, *The History of the Negro in Medicine,* p. 71; Hine, *Black Women in White,* p. 9.

51. Hine, *Black Women in White,* pp. 12–13; Sloan, "Early Black Nursing Schools and Responses of Black Nurses to their Educational Programs," p. 162.

52. Hine, *Black Women in White,* p. 20.

53. Ibid., p. xx; Morais, *The History of the Negro in Medicine,* p. 73.

54. Hine, *Black Women in White,* pp. 10–11, 20–21, 30–32, 46, 116–117.

55. Ibid., pp. 6, 9; Morais, *The History of the Negro in Medicine,* p. 70.

56. Sloan, "Early Black Nursing Schools and Responses of Black Nurses to their Educational Programs," p. 161.

57. Hine, *Black Women in White,* pp. 24–25, 76–77.

58. Ibid., pp. 103–104, 153.

59. Ibid., pp. 117–132, 148–150, 181–184, 188–192.

60. Ibid., p. 193.

61. See, for example, Shirley A. Vaughn Carter, "Reflections on Equal Edu-

cational Opportunity in Baccalaureate Nursing Programs," *Western Journal of Black Studies* 9 (Fall 1985): 152–157.

62. [Ebony Staff], "The Crisis of the Disappearing Black Hospitals," *Ebony* 47 (March 1992): 23–28.

63. For example, these processes of economic and cultural disruption are analyzed in John Sibley Butler, *Entrepreneurship and Self-Help among Black Americans: A Reconsideration of Race and Economics* (New York: State University of New York Press, 1991); Clovis E. Semmes, *Cultural Hegemony and African American Development* (Westport, Conn.: Praeger, 1992); Lerone Bennett, Jr., *Confrontation: Black and White* (Baltimore, Md.: Penguin Books, 1966); and E. Franklin Frazier, *Black Bourgeoisie: The Rise of a New Middle Class* (New York: Free Press, 1957).

64. See, for example, Margaret A. Rose, *The Post-Modern and the Post-Industrial: A Critical Analysis* (New York: Cambridge University Press, 1991).

65. The medical-industrial complex consists of medical technology and supply companies, pharmaceutical companies, hospitals and other types of medical care facilities, and physician and physician-related services. This sector of the economy is relatively monopolistic in that it is able to limit the legitimacy and use of competing health care systems, discourage self-care, and prohibit movement toward effective, low-cost, low-technology health care. Compare Arnold S. Relman, "The New Medical-Industrial Complex," *New England Journal of Medicine* 303 (October 23, 1980): 963–970.

66. See Victor R. Fuchs, *The Health Economy* (Cambridge, Mass.: Harvard University Press, 1986); Joshua M. Wiener, "Rationing in America: Overt and Covert," in Martin A. Strosberg, Joshua M. Wiener, Robert Baker, and I. Alan Fein, eds., *Rationing America's Medical Care: The Oregon Plan and Beyond* (Washington, D.C.: Brookings Institution, 1992), pp. 12–23.

67. The consumption of medical services and products always carries some negative result or risk, but radical consumption increases the negative returns considerably. See Ivan Illich, *Medical Nemesis: The Expropriation of Health* (New York: Pantheon, 1976); and Marcia Millman, *The Unkindest Cut: Life in the Backrooms of Medicine* (New York: William Morrow and Company, 1977).

68. Illich, *Medical Nemesis,* pp. 22–26.

69. Ibid., pp. 40–41; see also Lynn Payer, *Disease-Mongers: How Doctors, Drug Companies, and Insurers Are Making You Feel Sick* (New York: John Wiley and Son, 1992); and Mendelsohn, *Male Practice: How Doctors Manipulate Women.*

70. Illich, *Medical Nemesis,* pp. 32–33, 132–135, 216–217.

8

Contemporary Challenges to Health: Destabilization, Maladaptation, and Consumer Manipulation

The post-industrial period has brought together a confluence of factors that abnormally impede the goal of health. These are institutional destabilization, maladaptation, and consumer manipulation. Institutional destabilization is exemplified by the current post-industrial stresses on African-American family life. Chapter 4 noted that, for African Americans, in 1980 the number of female-headed families with children surpassed the number of married-couple families with children. The extended family, which could serve as a support to single-parent families, also declined. Because of historic oppression, a process of destabilization has always been part of the experience of African Americans, beginning with enslavement. However, post-industrial economic dislocation has intensified definite facets of this process and overwhelmed the resources of the African-American community to mitigate certain negative effects of historic inequality. The family is pivotal to the goal of health because of its role in providing and directing nutrition, caring and curing, and reducing stress. It is the leading institution of health because of its effect on lifestyle and its ability to insulate, protect, and invigorate its members. Religious and spiritual beliefs and values that may have positive implications for health also are reinforced through interactions in the family.

Maladaptation refers to health-destroying reactions and accommodations to changing social and environmental conditions. For example, traditional African-American dietary habits emerged from the formation of a slave culture that drew upon the limited availability of various food sources. Moreover, slavery introduced new substances into African-American consumption and new modes of thinking about one's self that were detrimental to African-American life. For example, for African

Americans: the recreational consumption of strong alcoholic drinks and tobacco as palliatives; the routine consumption of coffee, the propensity for large amounts of refined sugar, syrups, and fatty meats (primarily from pork); and for many, a limited use of vegetables and fruits are examples of maladaptive dietary practices rooted in slave culture. Other destructive maladaptations to oppression are the internalization of specific White-American cultural values and norms that demean African-American lives and create ambivalence and even hatred among African Americans about how they look. Profound insecurities over hair texture and length, skin color, and physiognomy heighten intraracial strife and psychological stress.[1]

Adaptation involves the interaction between structural (social organizational and resource-related) boundaries and an ethical system (a philosophy of right and wrong action) that directs accommodation to or gives guidance on how to alter those boundaries. An external system of oppression presents varying types of structural constraints and erects diverse methods of legitimation that make these constraints appear normal and justified. Internally a group may accept the definition and restrictions imposed by a system of oppression or it may challenge them. This process of discrimination is not either-or, however, and is complex and selective. Maladaptation resulting from oppression—in this case, a slave culture—can become central to identity and what are now normal patterns of sociability. To alter patterns of a slave culture that embody maladaptation, new cultural alternatives must emerge. As we have seen in Chapter 6, the possibilities for such change exists in indigenous (folk, popular, and alternative), yet evolving, health beliefs and practices.

Consumer manipulation is a key mediating dimension of health and is integrally connected to destabilization and maladaptation. Destabilization increases the ease of manipulation by reducing institutional and communal resistance. Maladaptations are also habits of consumption that become markets and sources of wealth for those who control production or who operate as mid-level suppliers. Shifts to more progressive forms of consumption could occur, but there is already inertia in habits, marketing, and production, which encourages the continuation of existing relations of consumption. Moreover, a post-industrial economic and cultural system tends to advocate radical consumption. The African-American community, which is habitually conditioned and coerced to accept the definitions and directives of a cultural system outside its own, cannot easily insulate itself from forces that prompt harmful consumption. The historic destruction and suppression of their own productive and self-defining capabilities, coupled with the intensive destabilization of the protective unit of the family, increases the health-related vulnerabilities of African Americans.

Nevertheless, African-American communities are not simply reactionary and impotent victims of these historic forces of oppression, which merely represent systemic tendencies and trends, albeit extremely crucial ones, that impede the collective development and welfare of African Americans. African Americans have always battled cultural and institutional assaults with varying degrees of success. If it were not for the strength and resiliency of this group, their health would probably be much worse. Thus, it is important to look within the African-American community to find the sources of strength that have contributed to survival and transcendence and magnify and preserve them.

NUTRITION AND STRESS

For African Americans, a crucial process that translates into added health problems is the interaction between stress and nutrition.

Common Nutritional Deficiencies

Generally speaking, the dietary and nutritional patterns of African Americans indicate certain inadequacies. African Americans at or near the poverty level typically consume diets that are marginal in vitamins A, B-complex, C, D, and E. They also consume insufficient amounts of the important minerals of calcium, magnesium, iron, and zinc.[2] One of every three Black Americans lives in poverty, compared to less than one of every eight White Americans.[3] In addition, regardless of socioeconomic status, many African Americans routinely consume diets low in complex carbohydrates and dietary fiber (fruits, vegetables, and whole grains).[4]

We also must pay attention to special nutritional requirements African Americans have that are related to genetic adaptations. For example, dark skin, which is presumably an adaptation to a sun-rich environment, does not synthesize vitamin D efficiently from the action of the sun on the skin. Vitamin D, among other things, is necessary to utilize calcium effectively. Moreover, a significant proportion of African Americans are lactose intolerant. This suggests that certain milk products are problematic as adequate sources of calcium and, if consumed in substantial amounts, may contribute to other health problems. Diets low in fresh fruits and vegetables add to possible calcium and magnesium deficiencies. The balance between calcium and magnesium is extremely important and necessary for the proper contraction and relaxation of muscles and the prevention of certain nervous afflictions.[5]

Older Black men and women particularly show greater deficiencies than Whites in the consumption of calories and potassium and in the consumption of vitamins A, B-complex, C, and D. Elderly African-American men and women are also more likely to skip meals.[6] An overreliance on eggs and fatty meats for breakfast and overcooking vegetables, which destroys important nutrients, may add to existing nutritional risks for the elderly.

Other risk factors that may restrict proper nutrition are mental confusion, poverty, physical disability, social isolation that results in the loss of interest in food, and inadequate knowledge regarding nutritionally balanced meals. Alcoholism, prescription and over-the-counter drugs, and bad teeth can also impair nutrition.[7]

Nutrition and Disease: The Case of Hypertension

Hypertension is an example of a disease entity and risk factor that has a relationship to nutrition. In addition, this condition is found much more frequently among Blacks than among Whites. Between the ages of 30 and 69, hypertension is half to two times more common in Blacks than in Whites. More severe forms of hypertension are five to seven times more common in Black men and women, respectively, when compared with their White counterparts. African Americans also experience disproportionately higher incidences of irreversible organ damage due to hypertension.[8]

Hypertension is defined as high, sustained blood pressure readings of at least 140 over 90.[9] It is a risk factor in coronary heart disease, stroke, and end-stage renal disease (destruction of kidney function).[10] We should emphasize, however, that slightly elevated blood pressure is a risk factor and not a disease. Telling people that they have hypertension when they do not creates undue anxiety and can make their health worse. Moreover, there is the issue of what blood pressure-reading should be considered high. A slight increase in the 140-over-90 standard can eliminate millions of people as prospects for blood pressure medication—something consumer-starved pharmaceutical companies resist. Drug therapy in some cases may have no benefit in extending the life of the patient and can produce other health problems. One also must be alert to the tendency by orthodox medical practitioners to exclude alternative drugless therapies (meditation, stress management, diet, and so on) that can reduce and control blood pressure. Other risk factors that can increase the dangers of high blood pressure should be considered when deciding to use drug therapy, which has accompanying side effects and risks.[11]

Hypertension is associated with a poor sodium-potassium balance. The daily sodium requirements of the body are very easy to meet, and many Americans frequently consume 8 to 40 times more sodium than they need on a day-to-day basis. Not only do people add salt to their food, they also consume processed foods that are high in sodium. Processing techniques tend to reduce the potassium content of foods. Hypertension is associated with diets higher than 6 grams of sodium per day, but it is associated even more highly with low potassium-sodium balance. Diets lacking in fresh fruits and vegetables are low in potassium relative to sodium. Blacks may not consume more sodium than Whites, but they consume less potassium relative to sodium. Moreover, a higher percentage of African Americans are salt sensitive. This may be a genetic predisposition related to the fact that Africans typically consumed high-potassium, low-sodium diets; African Americans may have adapted to lower levels of salt consumption.[12] Increased consumption of calcium and magnesium, of omega 6 and omega 3 polyunsaturated fatty acids, and of dietary fiber are associated with lowered blood pressure.[13]

Stress, Nutrition, and Biological Damage

In addition to the relationship between nutrition and disease, we need to include the supplemental role of stress. In fact, stress is also a notable component in the elevated blood pressure of African Americans.[14] In Chapters 1 and 3, I examined the significant role of stress as an agent in the disease process. Stress is normal and, in some cases, desirable, but when sustained for long periods of time without sufficient recovery or when extending beyond the resources (nutritional, biological, social, psychological, and the like) available to manage its destructive dimensions, negative health consequences abound.

I explained in Chapter 3 that various demands on the body produce the fight-or-flight, emergency response. A release of adrenal hormones prepares the body to confront impending difficulties. Blood pressure increases, the depth of breathing increases, sweating occurs, and the large muscles contract. Prolonged stress contributes to sodium and water retention and to reduced insulin production. Potassium—which is necessary for neural transmission and lowering the blood pressure—is lost. Other nutrients, which include vitamins A, the B complex, and C, are depleted. The body absorbs calcium, potassium, zinc, copper, and magnesium less efficiently. Stress tends to suppress the immune system, increasing susceptibility to disease and impeding the healing process. Repeated and prolonged stress can do physiological damage to important organs.[15]

The role of the B-complex vitamins and vitamin C are particularly important in the link between stress, organ damage, and chronic and degenerative diseases. The B-complex vitamins and vitamin C are water-soluble nutrients, and any excess is excreted through the urine. Since these vitamins are not stored to any appreciable degree, the body requires adequate supplies from the diet on a daily basis. Without understating the importance of other nutrients, the B-complex vitamins and vitamin C are probably the most critical components of the stress arousal response. The 13 or so B-complex vitamins and vitamin C work synergistically to provide the body with energy, converting carbohydrates into glucose and metabolizing fats and proteins. They are necessary for cortisol (secreted by adrenal glands) production and the normal functioning of the nervous system. The stress response creates an additional need for vitamin C and the B-complex vitamins, especially thiamine and riboflavin.[16]

Vitamin B1, or thiamine, for example, helps in the formation of hormones needed for relaxation, sleep, and pain reduction. It is essential for body growth and repair and to maintain the health of nerves, muscles, the heart, and the digestive system. Thiamine contributes to a good mental attitude. An absolute deficiency results in the disease beriberi, but inadequate supplies can lead to loss of appetite, irritability, emotional instability, lack of energy, difficulty digesting carbohydrates, muscle weakness, constipation, headaches, decreased attention span, chest pains, rapid heartbeat, cardiac damage, and heart failure. Excessive consumption of refined sugar, a common occurrence in this culture, can cause thiamine depletion. Consuming large amounts of candy and sugary carbonated drinks can produce symptoms similar to the early stages of beriberi. Nitrites and sulfites, baking soda, air pollutants, alcohol, some antibiotics, raw fish, coffee, and tea tend to interfere with absorption of thiamine. Smoking and drinking can deplete thiamine.[17]

Vitamin B2, or riboflavin, is needed to release energy from proteins and to aid in the synthesis of stress-related hormones, growth hormones, and insulin. It is essential to the growth, repair, and integrity of the nervous system. Deficiencies can cause loss of appetite; fatigue; digestive problems; anxiety; high blood pressure; lesions on the eyes, lips, mouth, genitals, or skin; cracks and sores in the corners of the mouth; a feeling of grit on the inside of the eyelids; burning of the eyes, eye fatigue, and dilation of the pupil; trembling; and other symptoms. Riboflavin is obstructed by oral contraceptives and certain antibiotics.[18]

As a whole, the B-complex vitamins generally are inadequately supplied in the diet. Processed foods as a rule lack these vitamins, and ingesting large quantities of refined sugar destroys them. Therefore, eating junk foods increases the need for B-complex vitamins but contributes very few of them. Alcohol destroys these vitamins, as do other substances like antibiotics, oral contraceptives, corticosteroids, aspirin, aspirin-related drugs, codeine, insecticides, and air pollutants. B-complex vitamins work together, and taking only one can induce a deficiency of the others. These vitamins are crucial to the stress response but also contribute to proper blood pressure, cholesterol, and glucose levels and to the health of the heart. The fact that they are not stored to any significant degree by the body but are needed daily highlights the importance of eating a diet rich in these nutrients.[19]

Vitamin C is similarly essential to the stress response; more of this nutrient is needed during stressful periods. It protects other vitamins and body tissues from injury by pollutants, poisons, and other destructive substances. Vitamin C assists the bacteria- and virus-fighting function of white blood cells and helps to lower serum cholesterol. It is important in the formation of red blood cells and in the maintenance of connective tissue. This water-soluble vitamin is needed daily and leaves the body in a few hours. It is used up quickly under stressful conditions and is depleted by tobacco smoke; high fever; prolonged ingestion of antibiotics, aspirin, and other pain killers; cortisone; and the inhalation of petroleum fumes. Deficiency symptoms include impaired digestion, bleeding gums, nosebleeds, lowered resistance to infection, slow healing of wounds and fractures, and shortness of breath.[20]

A number of food substances and consumables produce or mimic the stress arousal response in the body and are called, as a consequence, sympathomimetics. Caffeine, which is found in colas, coffee, tea, and chocolate, is a common example. It increases stress hormone secretion and therefore depletes the essential water soluble nutrients. Excessive salt intake can contribute to stress symptoms. Refined sugar intensifies the stress arousal response. Imprudent ingestion of large quantities of refined sugar can, after a short period of time, produce hypoglycemia and symptoms of anxiety, headaches, dizziness, rapid heartbeat, and irritability. Stress, therefore, has a profound relationship with a whole range of health-related habits. People may smoke or drink alcohol to avoid or adapt to stress. However, alcohol—besides its other destructive aspects—produces less tolerance to stress. The nicotine in cigarettes also stimulates the stress arousal response and is an addictive poison associated with withdrawal symptoms of headache, nausea, fatigue, and poor concentration.[21]

The effects of stress are extremely significant to the disease process and crucial, I believe, to understanding the disproportionately high morbidity and mortality that occur among African Americans. For example, it is clear that the same nutrients that are routinely insufficient in the diets of African Americans are also those that are secreted in greater quantities or poorly absorbed as a consequence of prolonged stress. Counterproductive consumption, which may include alcohol, drugs (over-the-counter, prescription, and illegal), empty calories from snacks and highly processed foods, large amounts of refined sugar, excessive salt, cigarettes, coffee, and the like destroy or deplete meager nutritional resources, which are needed to deal with the demands of prolonged stress. Missed meals and inadequate diets are also problems. Again, one-third of all African Americans live in poverty, and poverty is a major risk factor in poor nutrition. Moreover, we have known for some time that lower socioeconomic status correlates with higher stress and mortality.[22] One scholar who has examined this subject extensively observed, "There is no shortage of evidence that, as a target group, black Americans experience greater degrees of stressful life experiences than do their white counterparts."[23]

STRESS AND STATUS

Status is the degree of social worth afforded a person or group. When social status is lacking and there is a starvation for respect, stress increases. The stress response is heavily tied to the effects of hierarchy and domination. Research indicates that people who occupy a position of dominance are able to turn off the stress response more quickly. For subordinated (lower-status) groups, the stress response is more prolonged and harder to turn off. Poverty, therefore, is an important factor, but it is not decisive. The vertical status of individuals within a given social milieu and their sense of powerfulness or powerlessness, self-esteem, and coping ability mediate the stress response, and therefore its effects on the immune system and the health of vital organs.[24]

For African Americans, cultural hegemony involves an ecological arrangement that tends to reproduce negative hierarchies in all phases of life while weakening and overburdening the microinstitutions that are important to minimize and defend against stress. The family, of course, is a key protective institution, but in broader terms, any system of social support that helps to determine the quality of the microenvironment is significant.[25] The pockets of insulation and resiliency that have existed in the African-American community and are rooted in that group's culture have been essential to counteract the stress-related effects of structured inequality. They have not always been successful, but the overall results are commendable in light of U.S. history. Currently, economic dislocation and post-industrialism in the circumstances of enduring forces of cultural effacement create even more arduous obstacles to offsetting status-related stress. These comments by two researchers on the determinants of health are particularly relevant to African Americans in this day and age:

Unemployment, for example, may lead to illness (quite apart from its correlation with economic deprivation) if the unemployed individual becomes socially isolated and stigmatized. On the other hand, if support networks are in place to maintain social contacts, and if self-esteem is not undermined, then the health consequences may be minimal.[26]

STRESS, STATUS, AND HOMICIDE

An example of a major African-American public health problem that is related to stress (or distress) and the normative tendency of American society to devalue the social worth of African Americans is homicide. For African-American males, homicide is the third leading cause of death, and the rate is over six and a half times greater than the rate for White males. For African-American females, homicide is the eighth leading cause of death, and the rate is over three and a half times greater than the rate for

White females. Oppression has routinely spawned abnormally high homicide rates among African Americans, as revealed in tabulations that were
begun in 1914. Black-to-White ratios have been as high as 13-to-1 for
males and 8-to-1 for females. Ratios have declined from their highs in
1950, but there were sharp increases in rates in the 1960s and 1970s. Currently, African Americans make up about 12 percent of the population
but are approaching 50 percent of the murder victims. The most at-risk
group in the near past was African-American males 25 to 34 years of age,
but this category has become younger and is now the 15-to-24 age group.[27]

The sharp rise in the rate of deaths from homicide for African Americans corresponds to post-industrial economic dislocation and the added
strain on African-American family life. Rose and McClain emphasized an
issue that this volume has also addressed: African Americans did not gain
a foothold in the manufacturing economy of an industrializing nation. In
addition, African-American males, more than any other group, were inadequately positioned to make the transition from an industrial society to
a post-industrial one.[28] Rose and McClain have argued persuasively that
the rise in the risk of homicide corresponded with structural changes in
the urban economy:

One of the primary negative externalities associated with the spread of post-
industrialism is a heightened risk of violent victimization. The elevation of risk is
manifested most often in those sub-areas of the city in which exclusion from participation in the new economy is most evident, especially if the excluded individuals represent first-time labor force entrants.[29]

These researchers also advanced the argument that there is an added
interaction between structure and culture. Post-industrial society has made
the mass media a pervasive and powerful socializing institution. Violence
on television (and, I would argue, through other media—movies and music
lyrics, for example) has altered American culture as youth imitate destructive behavior that has been glamorized.[30]

A culture of violence is not new to American society, however. Sociologist Robert Staples made the point that African-American violence is
a part of the normative pattern of violence in the United States. The
frontier violence used in the founding of this country is an example. However, society makes the distinction between legitimate and illegitimate violence. American popular culture glorifies violence and the gun as means
of achieving respect. Furthermore, frustration and powerlessness breed
violence. The frustrations of economic dislocation correspond to increased
spousal violence and child abuse, and economic problems especially make
single parenthood more stressful. Moreover, the misdirected frustration of
oppression can surface in self-destructive ways. Rape, Staples explained,
is an aggressive act against females, which also may be an externalization

of social repression resulting from barriers to normal expressions of man-hood.[31] Excessive homicide rates among African Americans, therefore, are a form of maladaptation to ecological stress.

Violence and homicide are also related to the growth of illegal econo-mies, most specifically, the sale of cocaine and crack cocaine. For example, cocaine-related emergency room episodes for African-American males in-creased from 8,159 in 1985 to 46,064 in 1992; for African-American fe-males, the increase was from 3,959 to 22,187.[32] Illegal economies are outcomes of the fact that some economically dispossessed people will seek alternative types of economic activity to meet what they perceive as their social needs. Economic dislocation contributes to illegal economies, but the post-industrial culture of radical materialism is an added impetus for maladaptation. We are taught, in an overproduced society, that our human worth is tied to the acquisition of material goods. This combination of structural and cultural aberrations is most detrimental to people who are starved for respect and economically disadvantaged.

Violence connected to drug trafficking is the result of economic com-petition over markets and other business-related disputes.[33] Increased vi-olence is understandable if we recognized that disputes involving illegal activity cannot be settled by an established legal authority. History has already given us a model of the violence that can come from the unre-gulated and illegal sale of a drug for which there is substantial demand, which comes from the drug's addictive qualities as well as from its com-mercial potential. That model was the organized crime activity and gang wars that characterized the era of Prohibition and the illegal sale of al-cohol. In fact, African-American youth who engage in illegal drug econ-omies have looked to the media glorification of organized crime and gangsterism as the model for their behavior. Drive-by shootings, the in-discriminate use of automatic weapons, and ruthlessness are key compo-nents of maladaptive responses to American cultural values—the pursuit of material gain, notoriety, and respect through vicious competition and violence.

Darnell Hawkins has also emphasized the role of American values in promoting African-American homicide. He disclosed that legal and social controls have tended to devalue Black life as a social norm. Historically, African Americans have been punished severely for killing Whites but not other Blacks (also, Whites were not punished at all, in many cases, for killing Blacks), and unequal legal sanctions encourage violence as a form of conflict resolution within a group that has learned to devalue itself. Hawkins also points to the ecological stress of economic dislocation and explains that violence represents an effort to gain control in light of po-litical, economic, and social disadvantage. Excessive intragroup violence is also a maladaptive expression of frustration spawned by inequality.[34]

American cultural values have always encouraged African Americans to demean other African Americans and heighten the potential for star-vation for respect. Hylan Lewis revealed the structural basis for this ten-dency in his classic study, *Blackways of Kent.* He showed that respect was an important value for African Americans but that racial inequality cre-ated a situation where the disrespect African Americans routinely had to tolerate from mainstream White America resulted, in too many cases, in an extreme lack of tolerance of slights from other Blacks. He explained:

Practically every Negro in this bi-racial situation tends to be respect-starved. When the opportunity affords, he will demand it, or satisfy his need for it [respect] in-directly or subtly, when whites are involved; the use of direct aggression varies with the person and the situation. Consistent with this "having to take it" is the Negro's behavior within his own group: it is the one place where he doesn't have to "take it." Aggressiveness and querulousness are symptomatic of a respect-starved group; they have a cumulative and persistent quality insofar as "touchiness begets touchiness."[35]

Lewis also explains that the African Americans he studied used friendli-ness, courtesy, and kindness to break through barriers of extreme sensi-tivity.[36] Extending respect, regardless of status, was exceptionally important to transcend the effects of racial inequality and subordination.

Homicides most often occur between family and friends and within one's own racial/ethnic group. Whites generally kill Whites and Blacks generally kill Blacks, but African-American deaths are excessive. Exces-sive violence and homicide are tied to structural and cultural barriers that spawn maladaptation to inequality and mainstream American values. An increased use of firearms is associated with nearly all increases in homi-cide; alcohol use is also an important factor.[37] Institutional destabilization, which is connected to inequality and economic dislocation, increases stress and distress. Even consumer manipulation comes into play when one con-siders that the glorification of violence, gangsterism, and the gun are part of a process of commercial exploitation. The extremes of graphic violence are used by the media to capture the attention of consumers in an over-produced marketplace.

DISEASES OF LIFESTYLE AND CONSUMPTION

Similarly, the conditions created by structured inequality exacerbate chronic and degenerative diseases among African Americans, as they did for infectious diseases when this type of health problem predominated among the population. Such leading causes of death and major risk factors that disproportionately affect African Americans as heart disease and stroke, cancer, diabetes, obesity, infant mortality, alcohol consumption, smoking cigarettes, and the like are deeply connected to complex social and historical factors that affect how African Americans live and consume. AIDS, like tuberculosis and syphilis in an earlier era, is also found disproportionately among African Americans because of continuing relationships of inequality. The socially induced dependency of post-industrialism and cultural hegemony creates added barriers to the goal of health through their impact on consumption and key socializing and protective institutions.

Cerebrovascular and Coronary Heart Disease

Cerebrovascular disease (stroke) is the third leading cause of death for African Americans and accounts for more excess deaths than any other disease when compared to White Americans.[38] The major risk factors are hypertension, abnormal blood lipids (high cholesterol), and smoking. We have already examined related nutritional factors in hypertension. Stress is also a critical factor in hypertension, and hypertension is a prime stimulus for stroke in African Americans.[39] The evidence suggests that environment has a strong effect on hypertension since Africans in rural areas tend not to have hypertension, while movement to urban areas increases incidence of the condition. Moreover, African Americans show patterns of diseased cerebral blood vessels that are closer to those of Whites in the United States than to West Africans.[40]

Diseases of the heart, as they are for all Americans, are the leading cause of death for African Americans. The death rates are much higher for Black Americans than for White Americans, despite significant declines for both groups over the years.[41] The cardiac disorder that is of most concern results from inadequate circulation of the blood to adjacent areas of the heart muscle. This impeded blood flow is generally caused by a narrowing of the coronary arteries, a process known as atherosclerosis, which is a disease process that can last for decades before the onset of symptoms. It consists of a loss of elasticity and a thickening of the inner portion of the blood vessel, which can eventually lead to blockage. When the heart function is affected, the condition is called coronary heart disease.[42]

The major risk factors in coronary heart disease are obesity, smoking, high cholesterol levels, and hypertension. The effects of hypertension are not clear, however, since some populations of Blacks (Africans and Caribbeans) exhibit a high incidence of hypertension but a low incidence of coronary heart disease.[43] Elevated levels of serum cholesterol and low-density lipoprotein cholesterol (LDL-C) are associated with atherosclerosis. A high intake of saturated fat is the major risk factor for abnormal serum cholesterol and LDL-C. The dietary intake of cholesterol has a less significant effect on serum cholesterol levels. Abdominal fat increases the risk of coronary heart disease.[44] Higher levels of high-density lipoprotein cholesterol (HDL-C) are associated with lowered risk of coronary heart disease. Saturated fats tend to raise cholesterol, while polyunsaturated fats tend to lower cholesterol levels; monounsaturated fats are neutral. Consuming fish oils and maintaining a diet high in fiber tends to lower cholesterol levels, as does the substitution of vegetable protein for animal protein.[45]

Since there is no clear overall difference in the serum cholesterol levels of Blacks and Whites or in the percent of total calories the two groups consume from fat, one must focus more on the probable interactions of multiple risk factors in coronary heart disease (there are, however, some indications that African Americans consume higher levels of fat and suffer from higher levels of cholesterol). Critical multiple risk factors are stress, hypertension, and obesity. Being overweight is particularly problematic for African-American women. Between the ages of 20 and 74, nearly half of all African-American women are overweight. African Americans consume poorer diets and receive fewer of the protective benefits of certain foods. At the same time, status-induced stress increases the need for certain nutrients, necessitating greater nutritional density.[46]

Cancer

Cancer is the second leading cause of death in the United States and among African Americans. Again, the death rates for African Americans are much higher than for White Americans and the survival rates are lower; for all cancers, Blacks have a 10 percent higher incidence and a 30 percent higher mortality.[47] Various cancers are strongly associated with diet, smoking, alcohol consumption, and socioeconomic status.[48] Lung cancer is associated with smoking, and smoking and drinking alcohol work synergistically to increase the risk of cancers of the mouth, larynx, and esophagus. The abuse of alcohol is also associated with poor nutrition, and alcoholism depletes various essential and protective nutrients.[49] Breast, colon, and prostate cancers are correlated with high fat consumption and being overweight. Drinking alcohol is also a risk factor for breast cancer. The incidence of cancer of the cervix increases with body weight, and salt-cured, salt-pickled, and smoked foods are highly associated with stomach and esophageal cancers.[50]

The incidence of all these cancers tends to decline as fruit and vegetable consumption goes up and with other dietary adjustments. High-fiber diets are associated with lower amounts of colon cancer. Moreover, foods high in vitamin A and beta carotene appear to protect against cancer. For example, cruciferous vegetables like cabbage, broccoli, brussels sprouts, and cauliflower are very good anticancer agents. There is the possibility that other unknown factors in these foods, rather than a single vitamin, may fight cancer. Foods containing vitamins C, E, and the trace mineral selenium appear to minimize the formation of carcinogens.[51] Current research suggests that African Americans should reduce fat (for example, eliminate red meat and shift from animal protein to vegetable protein sources) to 30 percent or less of calories; increase fiber (eat whole grains and whole-grain products) to 20 to 30 grams daily; eat a variety and substantial quantity of fresh fruits and vegetables daily; abstain from alcohol, tobacco, and illicit drugs; and avoid added salt and sugar, obesity, empty calorie (junk) foods that lack naturally occurring nutrients, and salt-cured, salt-pickled, and smoked foods.[52]

Diabetes and Obesity

Diabetes is one of the most significant health problems among African Americans and further documents the crucial importance of the convergence of environmental, social, and cultural factors that affect health. It is one of the six health categories that collectively account for over 80 percent of all excess deaths among African Americans. (Heart disease and stroke, homicide and accidents, cancer, infant mortality, and cirrhosis are the other five.)[53] Diabetes is more common among women than men and more common among Blacks than Whites. It is the tenth leading cause of death for African-American males and the fourth leading cause of death for African-American females.[54] Poverty and lower educational attainment are associated with diabetes, but obesity is the most powerful risk factor in the most prevalent form of the disease.[55]

Diabetes is itself a risk factor for coronary heart disease and stroke and for very serious complications, which include blindness, the need for amputation of limbs, and destruction of kidney function. Diabetes may lead to retinopathy, a condition in which the capillaries swell and hemorrhage within the retina and impair portions of the eye that are needed for clear vision. Diabetes is the leading cause of blindness for persons 20 to 74 years of age. It contributes to peripheral arterial disease, which impairs normally elastic arterial walls, causing them to harden and develop internal deposits of plaque; gangrene and ulceration may require the amputation of limbs. Diabetes may cause the cleaning function of the kidneys to slowly degenerate (diabetic nephropathy), since high blood sugar forces the kidneys to filter more blood than needed. Because of the associated complications and risk factors, diabetes has a much more profound impact on health and mortality than standard health-related statistics indicate.[56]

Diabetes mellitus is a "chronic systemic disease characterized by glucose intolerance or the inability of the body to properly use glucose."[57] Either the pancreas does not produce enough insulin (the hormone necessary to metabolize blood sugar and maintain the proper blood sugar level) or it produces none at all; alternately, the cells of the body do not receive insulin appropriately and the ability to use insulin is impaired.[58]

There are two principal types of diabetes. Type I (insulin-dependent) diabetes can occur at any age but usually occurs in children. It is less common in Blacks than Whites and affects 5 to 10 percent of the known diabetic population. Type II (non–insulin dependent) diabetes can occur at any age but appears most often among adults over 40. It is more common among Blacks than Whites and affects 90 to 95 percent of the known diabetic population. There are other types of diabetes—for example, gestational, which occurs during pregnancy—but Type II diabetes is the most widespread and most strongly associated with social factors.[59]

The relationship of Type II diabetes to obesity and its disproportionate impact on African-American women is pronounced. Studies have indicated that two-thirds to nine-tenths of individuals with Type II diabetes may be classified as obese at the time of diagnosis. The disease correlates highly with individuals who weigh more than 25 percent over their ideal body weight. The occurrence of obesity among African-American women when compared to White women is extreme, reaching a high of 50 percent for ages 55 to 64.[60] An added factor in the obesity equation is that a greater waist to hip ratio is associated with a higher incidence of Type II diabetes.[61] Moreover, regardless of insulin output, obesity tends to hamper the body's ability to use insulin.[62] In the United States, the risk of dying from diabetes mellitus for Black women is over two and a half times greater than the risk for White women.[63]

Being overweight and obese are complex issues related to energy balance, dietary and nutritional patterns, and a host of other social and biological factors. We should avoid blaming the victim and oversimplifying this important health issue. African-American women are under intense stress from multiple social factors related to inequality and economic dislocation. Current social forces tend to fracture relationships between African-American men and women, disrupt self-esteem, and subvert microprocesses that govern positive health behavior. As a consequence, even though Type II diabetes is strongly associated with obesity, obesity is itself an indicator of other social patterns that need to be reconfigured.[64]

Infant Mortality

Infant mortality is another urgent health issue facing African Americans that is strongly related to multiple social and environmental factors influenced by structured inequality. Despite the fact that infant mortality has declined dramatically in this century for all groups, the gap between Blacks and Whites has widened, to the extent that today, infant mortality rates for Blacks are twice those for Whites.[65] The key to a healthy child is a healthy mother, but in this day and age, infant mortality has become complicated by maternal substance abuse. Tobacco, alcohol, and other drugs, which include cocaine, heroin, methadone, phencyclidine hydrochloride

(PCP), and others, place the life of the mother and newborn in jeopardy. If the child survives, the effects of maternal substance abuse can have far-reaching effects on future development and life chances. Substance abuse—especially by mothers involved in intravenous drug use—is associated with perinatal AIDS and congenital syphilis. Cigarettes, alcohol, and illegal drug use increase the risk of a low-birth-weight child, and low birth weight is the most potent correlate of infant mortality.[66]

The relationship of low birth weight to infant mortality is striking. A low-birth-weight infant—a newborn weighing less than 5.5 pounds (2,500 grams)—is 40 times more likely than an infant of average weight to die in the first month. A very low-birth-weight infant—a newborn weighing less than 3.3 pounds (1,500 grams)—is 200 times more likely to die in the first month. African Americans have the highest percentage of low-birth-weight babies of all U.S. ethnic groups. The Black low-birth-weight rate is over twice the White rate, and the Black very low-birth-weight rate is over three times the White rate.[67]

Low birth weight is associated with a number of risk factors, but the confluence of logical and empirical evidence point to elements that affect the nutritional and biological integrity of the mother before and during pregnancy. Prenatal care tends to reduce the incidence of low birth weight and infant mortality.[68] However, a best weight has not been definitively established, and small Black infants have a better survival rate than small White infants. Moreover, Black-White differences in low birth weight and in infant mortality have been found to be greater in low-risk women than in high-risk women.[69] Low-risk Blacks probably experience poorer overall social and environmental factors than their White counterparts, which may not be easily negated by certain intervention strategies. Moreover, adaptive patterns may exist that tend to protect Black low-birth-weight infants under certain conditions.[70] Prenatal care, no doubt, is most effective if it results in improved nutrition, relevant lifestyle change (for example, proper exercise and rest; cessation of smoking, alcohol consumption, and drug use; and so on), and social support capable of reducing stress and reinforcing positive health behaviors.[71] Understanding how prenatal care and social support affect young mothers, and not focusing on the simple fact of age, is probably most important in lowering infant mortality among adolescent mothers.[72] Clearly, though, negative lifestyle factors, lower socioeconomic status, and poor environmental conditions do highly correlate with lower birth weight and higher infant mortality.[73]

The importance of nutrition and biological integrity are further supported by the fact that pre-pregnancy weight and adequate weight gain during pregnancy are important determinants of healthy infants, even though an optimum weight has not been defined. Obesity, for example, significantly increases maternal complications. Environmental racism is another factor. Lead poisoning is a significant health issue for African-

Americans and is linked to historic patterns of institutional racism. Maternal exposure to lead can increase the risk of low-birth-weight babies and bolster infant mortality.[74] The convergence of distinctive and unique social and environmental factors that affect African-American health are clearly at work in African-American infant mortality.

Drugs and Consumer Manipulation

It is no accident that drugs and consumer manipulation go hand in hand, as each symbolizes the other. The struggle to release the inhibition to buy while creating dependency has found an important tool in the drug. The drug is addictive, or at least habit forming. It is easy to consume and contributes to passivity. If a drug can be claimed as a remedy, the only goal is to consume. Of course, there are drugs that are useful and, in some instances, necessary, but one can cross the line from need to want very easily. Indeed, the seller of the drug will always say that consumers need the drug and that it will make them better in some way. Given the size of the legitimate and illegitimate market for drugs—both medicinal and social—it is easy to conclude that American society is a drug culture. The buyer must be aware and have the power to discriminate and to impose restraint; there must be alternatives to consuming the drug, and the consumer must not have lost the will to act.

There is not much difference in the approaches to marketing legal and illicit drugs. A crack cocaine dealer provides a free sample to whomever he or she hopes is a potential customer. Similarly, a model from an ad agency passes out free samples for a particular brand of cigarettes on a busy street corner. Both sellers seek to obtain market share. The cigarette company, of course, is backed by law and social legitimacy. It can openly hire others to market and distribute. Each seller is aware of the social costs and the addictiveness of the products.

All Americans must confront merchants of misery hidden behind the facade of pleasure, but some must confront this phenomenon more than others, and without protective resources. The power and awareness required are exactly the qualities that American society tends to deny African Americans. The results, in terms of health and well-being, are devastating.

White Americans, for example, consume more alcohol and drink more heavily than Blacks, but African Americans are overrepresented in most indirect measures of alcohol problems like cirrhosis and esophageal cancer. Alcohol may be the greatest contributor to the poor health of African Americans because of its multiple and interconnected injurious consequences. It makes diseases worse, and it has a major role in homicide and other crimes, automobile injuries and deaths, family violence, fetal alcohol syndrome (caused by pregnant women who drink, it leads to retardation),

birth defects, risk for contracting AIDS, unwanted pregnancies, delin-
quency, and school failure.[75] We have already examined alcohol's destructive effects on nutrition and counterproductive role in managing stress.

Contrary to public perception, young White males are more likely to
use illegal drugs than young Black males, and there is little overall difference in illegal drug use between Black and White Americans. Blacks have
less involvement with cocaine, but young Blacks have higher rates of heroin use. Crack cocaine, which is more addictive than powdered cocaine,
is found more frequently in urban than rural and suburban areas.[76] In the
same way that African Americans are not major producers and distributors of goods in the general economy, they are not major producers and
distributors of alcohol, tobacco, or illegal drugs. African Americans have
been targeted and cultivated as consumers—going back to the time of
slavery—and they are frequently encouraged to use the most potent and
addictive form of a given drug. Socially induced powerlessness, maladaptation, and ignorance facilitates the process.

AIDS is a prime example of how a disease can disproportionately affect
a community when it is subject to systemic institutional destabilization. Its
impact is similar to the destructive paths of tuberculosis and syphilis when
there were no cures for these diseases. Poverty, powerlessness, ignorance,
and intravenous drug use exacerbate the spread of AIDS. It is primarily
a blood-borne disease, and conditions of poor health that contribute to
lesions or breaks in the skin assist in the spread of the disease when contact is made with the blood of an infected person. White bisexual and
homosexual men remain the largest at-risk group, but AIDS cases and
deaths are grossly overrepresented among African Americans. Blacks
aged 13 years and older at the time of diagnosis represent well over 30
percent of the AIDS deaths annually. Black females aged 13 years and
older and Black children under 13 are approaching 60 percent of the
deaths in their respective categories. If a female intravenous drug user or
a female sexual partner of an intravenous drug user becomes pregnant,
she is at high risk for AIDS and for infecting her fetus or newborn. As a
consequence, AIDS is rapidly becoming a major factor in infant and child
mortality.[77]

Tobacco, like certain potent alcoholic beverages, was introduced to Africans during slavery as a palliative and controlling agent; today, it is a
major source of morbidity and mortality for all Americans, and for African
Americans in particular. Tobacco kills 390,000 people in the United States
annually and is responsible for one of every six deaths. It is a major risk
factor in diseases of the heart and blood vessels; chronic bronchitis and
emphysema; and cancers of the lung, larynx, pharynx, oral cavity, esophagus, pancreas, and bladder; and in respiratory infections and stomach
ulcers. Smoking causes almost 90 percent of all lung cancer deaths and 30

percent of all cancer deaths. Smokers are more likely to be overweight and consume poorer diets.[78]

Smoking hurts many innocent and vulnerable people. Passive smoke causes lung cancer and other diseases in nonsmokers. This smoke normally contains at least 43 chemical compounds that are carcinogenic and some that are mutagenic—they can cause possible harmful changes to the genetic materials of cells. Smoking contributes to 20 to 30 percent of low-birth-weight babies. Exposing children to passive smoke induces serious respiratory problems such as asthma and increases hospitalizations for bronchitis, pneumonia, and ear infections. Passive smoke can create lung problems in children that extend into adulthood. Smoking, the most preventable cause of death, is declining among adults in this country, but disproportionately fewer Blacks than Whites are giving up smoking. Blacks are smoking stronger cigarettes, and young people continue to pick up the debilitating habit. Moreover, smoking is increasingly becoming a practice of the less educated segments of the society.[79]

Producers, distributors, and marketers of drugs and other health-destroying products have long recognized the potential of African American communities as vulnerable consumers. Sociologist E. Franklin Frazier noted long ago that the marketing of cigarettes, alcoholic beverages, and soft drinks to African Americans was one of the earliest opportunities for Black employment in the private sector.[80] Status-induced stress, poverty, and structured inequality create a ready market for palliatives. African Americans watch significantly more television than the general population. They are very responsive to culturally sensitive advertising, and corporations that sell alcoholic beverages and cigarettes (also fast foods and soft drinks) take advantage of this. African-American magazines are overly dependent on cigarette and alcohol advertising since other large advertisers frequently overlook Black-owned publications. Furthermore, there are disproportionate numbers of liquor and "party" stores and excessive billboards advertising cigarettes and alcohol in African-American communities. Cigarette and alcoholic beverage companies sponsor cultural and artistic groups and events by Blacks and give money to Black-oriented scholarship funds in order to gain name recognition and consumer trust. Moreover, African-American elites who manage Black-oriented Civil Rights and philanthropic agencies develop close relationships with cigarette, liquor, fast food, and soft drink companies and deliver to them the goodwill and buying power of the African-American community.[81]

SUMMARY AND CONCLUSION

In sum, the interaction of inequality and post-industrialism places an added burden on the health of African Americans. Inequality tends to produce disproportionate institutional destabilization, cultural maladaptation, and consumer manipulation. Post-industrialism heightens external forces of consumer manipulation, which promote harmful health results. At the same time, however, institutional destabilization (most notably, of the family) weakens the ability to resist and reshape adverse forces of consumer manipulation. Furthermore, a crucial mediating factor in the health process is the interaction between various forms of stress and nutrition. Historic and contemporary inequality stimulates additional stress (for example, status-induced stress, environmental racism, assaults on self-esteem, respect starvation, poverty, economic dislocation, and so on), which interacts with maladaptive patterns of consumption to lower the biological integrity of African Americans. Thus, increased collective power and a heightened health consciousness are central to their well-being.

In the next chapter we will explore possible solutions to African-American health needs.

NOTES

1. See, for example, Darlene Powell Hopson and Derek S. Hopson, *Different and Wonderful: Raising Black Children in a Race-Conscious Society* (New York: Simon and Schuster, 1992); Clovis E. Semmes, *Cultural Hegemony and African American Development* (Westport, Conn.: Praeger, 1992), pp. 93–110.

2. Deborah E. Blocker, "Nutritional Concerns of Black Americans," in Ivor Lensworth Livingston, ed., *Handbook of Black American Health: The Mosaic of Conditions, Issues, Policies, and Prospects* (Westport, Conn.: Greenwood Press, 1994), p. 269.

3. See United States, National Center for Health Statistics, *Health, United States 1993* (Hyattsville, Md.: Public Health Service, 1994), p. 63.

4. Blocker, "Nutritional Concerns of Black Americans," p. 269.

5. See Kenneth F. Kiple and Virginia Himmelsteib King, *Another Dimension to the Black Diaspora: Diet, Disease, and Racism* (New York: Cambridge University Press, 1981), pp. 195–200; Nutrition Search, Inc., *Nutrition Almanac*, rev. ed. (New York: McGraw-Hill, 1979), pp. 63–64, 73–74.

6. Norge W. Jerome, "Dietary Intake and Nutritional Status of Older U.S. Blacks: An Overview," in James S. Jackson, ed., *The Black American Elderly: Research on Physical and Psychosocial Health* (New York: Springer, 1988), pp. 137–139.

7. Ibid., pp. 140–142.

8. United States, *Health, United States 1993*, p. 164; Ivor Lensworth Livingston, "Stress, Hypertension and Renal Disease in Black Americans: A Review with Implications," *National Journal of Sociology* 5 (Fall 1991): 146–147.

9. Ibid.

10. National Research Council Committee on the Status of Black Americans, *A Common Destiny: Blacks and American Society* (Washington, D.C.: National Academy Press, 1989), p. 422; Blocker, "Nutritional Concerns of Black Americans," p. 272.

11. See Lynn Payer, *Disease-Mongers: How Doctors, Drug Companies, and In-*

surers Are Making You Feel Sick (New York: John Wiley and Son, 1992), pp. 32, 181–182; George Berkley, *On Being Black and Healthy: How Black Americans Can Lead Longer and Healthier Lives* (Englewood Cliffs, N.J.: Prentice-Hall, 1982), p. 20.

12. Berkley, *On Being Black and Healthy,* pp. 31–34; Blocker, "Nutritional Concerns of Black Americans," p. 272; Norman B. Anderson, "Aging and Hypertension among Blacks: A Multidimensional Perspective," in James S. Jackson, *The Black American Elderly: Research on Physical and Psychosocial Health* (New York: Springer, 1988), pp. 190–214.

13. Blocker, "Nutritional Concerns of Black Americans," p. 272.

14. Ivor Lensworth Livingston, "Stress, Hypertension and Renal Disease in Black Americans," p. 151.

15. See Donald R. Morse and Robert L. Pollack, *Nutrition, Stress, and Aging: A Holistic Approach to the Relationship among Stress and Food Selection, Digestion, Nutrients, Body Weight, Disease, and Longevity* (New York: AMS Press, 1988); Jonathan Smith, *Understanding Stress and Coping* (New York: Macmillan, 1993); Dorothy H. G. Cotton, *Stress Management: An Integrated Approach to Therapy* (New York: Brunner/Mazel, 1990), pp. 175–176.

16. Nutrition Search, Inc., *Nutrition Almanac,* pp. 18–24; Smith, *Understanding Stress and Coping,* p. 137; Cotton, *Stress Management,* p. 175.

17. Nutrition Search, Inc., *Nutrition Almanac,* pp. 21–22; Morse and Pollack, *Nutrition, Stress, and Aging,* pp. 86–87.

18. Nutrition Search, Inc., *Nutrition Almanac,* p. 24; Morse and Pollack, *Nutrition, Stress, and Aging,* p. 87.

19. Smith, *Understanding Stress and Coping,* p. 137; Morse and Pollack, *Nutrition, Stress, and Aging,* pp. 79–92.

20. Morse and Pollack, *Nutrition, Stress, and Aging,* pp. 80–83; Nutrition Search, Inc., *Nutrition Almanac,* pp. 43–44.

21. Smith, *Understanding Stress and Coping,* pp. 137, 139; Cotton, *Stress Management,* p. 176.

22. See for example, Monroe Learner, "Social Differences in Physical Health," in John Kosa and Irving Kenneth Zola, eds., *Poverty and Health: A Sociological Analysis* (Cambridge, Mass.: Harvard University Press, 1975), pp. 80–134; Marc Fried, "Social Differences in Mental Health," in John Kosa and Irving Kenneth Zola, eds., *Poverty and Health: A Sociological Analysis* (Cambridge, Mass.: Harvard University Press, 1975), p. 189.

23. Ivor Lensworth Livingston, "Stress, Hypertension and Renal Disease in Black Americans," p. 151.

24. See Robert G. Evans, "Introduction," in Robert G. Evans, Morris L. Barer, and Theodore R. Marmor, eds., *Why Are Some People Healthy and Others Not? The Determinants of Health of Populations* (New York: Aldine DeGruyter, 1994), pp. 5–15.

25. Ibid., pp. 19–23.

26. Robert G. Evans and G. L. Stoddart, "Producing Health, Consuming Health Care," in Robert G. Evans, Morris L. Baer, and Theodore R. Marmor, eds. *Why Are Some People Healthy and Others Not? The Determinants of Health of Populations* (New York: Aldine DeGruyter, 1994), p. 52.

27. United States, *Health, United States 1993,* pp. 93–94, 97–98, 130; Wornie L.

Reed, *The Health and Medical Care of African-Americans* (Boston: University of Massachusetts at Boston, William Monroe Trotter Institute, 1992), pp. 55, 57–59.

28. Harold M. Rose and Paula D. McClain, *Race, Place, and Risk: Black Homicide in Urban America* (Albany: State University of New York Press, 1990), pp. 4, 139; see also Reed, *The Health and Medical Care of African-Americans*, pp. 57–59.

29. Ibid., p. 241.

30. Ibid., p. 243.

31. Robert Staples, "The Masculine Way of Violence," in Darnell F. Hawkins, ed., *Homicide among Black Americans* (Lanham, Md.: University Press of America, 1986), pp. 137–152.

32. United States, *Health, United States 1993*, p. 162.

33. National Research Council on the Committee on the Status of Black Americans, *A Common Destiny: Blacks and American Society*, pp. 461–463.

34. Darnell F. Hawkins, "Black and White Homicide Differentials: Alternatives to an Inadequate Theory," in Darnell F. Hawkins, ed., *Homicide among Black Americans* (Lanham, Md.: University Press of America, 1986), pp. 114–120, 124–125.

35. Hylan Lewis, *Blackways of Kent* (New Haven, Conn.: College and University Press, 1964), p. 221.

36. Ibid.

37. Reed, *The Health and Medical Care of African-Americans*, pp. 59–62.

38. Gary H. Friday, "Cerebrovascular Disease in Blacks," in Ivor Lensworth Livingston, ed., *Handbook of Black American Health: The Mosaic of Conditions, Issues, Policies, and Prospects* (Westport, Conn.: Greenwood Press, 1994), p. 33; United States, *Health, United States 1993*, pp. 97–98.

39. Carolyn J. Hildreth and Elijah Sanders, "Heart Disease, Stroke, and Hypertension in Blacks," in Ronald L. Braithwaite and Sandra E. Taylor, eds., *Health Issues in the Black Community* (San Francisco: Jossey-Bass, 1992), p. 90.

40. Friday, "Cerebrovascular Disease in Blacks," pp. 39–40.

41. United States, *Health, United States 1993*, pp. 93–94.

42. C. Everett Koop, *The Surgeon General's Report on Nutrition and Health 1988* (Rocklin, Calif.: Prima Publishing and Communications, 1989), p. 83; Charles Curry, "Coronary Artery Disease in Blacks," in Ivor Lensworth Livingston, ed., *Handbook of Black American Health: The Mosaic of Conditions, Issues, Policies, and Prospects* (Westport, Conn.: Greenwood Press, 1994), pp. 24–32.

43. Ibid., p. 27.

44. Blocker, "Nutritional Concerns of Black Americans," pp. 270–271.

45. Koop, *The Surgeon General's Report of Nutrition and Health*, pp. 107–109.

46. United States, *Health, United States 1993*, pp. 165, 167; Ki Moon Bang, "Cancer and Black Americans," in Ivor Lensworth Livingston, ed., *Handbook of Black American Health: The Mosaic of Conditions, Issues, Policies, and Prospects* (Westport, Conn.: Greenwood Press, 1994), p. 86.

47. Berkley, *On Being Black and Healthy*, p. 47; United States, *Health, United States 1993*, pp. 93–94.

48. Bang, "Cancer and Black Americans," pp. 81, 85–88.

49. Koop, *The Surgeon General's Report on Nutrition and Health*, p. 214.

50. Ibid., p. 223.

51. Ibid., pp. 210. 213, 217–219.

52. Ibid., p. 192; there are multiple ways to achieve better nutrition. The African-American community needs specific nutritional guidelines in light of its unique health-related circumstances.

53. Reed, *The Health and Medical Care of African-Americans.* p. 5; Frederick G. Murphy and Joycelyn M. Elders, "Diabetes and the Black Community," in Ronald L. Braithwaite and Sandra E. Taylor, eds., *Health Issues in the Black Community* (San Francisco: Jossey-Bass, 1992), p. 121.

54. United States, *Health, United States 1993,* pp. 97–98.

55. Koop, *The Surgeon General's Report on Nutrition and Health 1988,* p. 256; Leslie Lieberman, "Diabetes and Obesity in Elderly Black Americans," in James S. Jackson, ed., *The Black American Elderly: Research on Physical and Psychosocial Health* (New York: Springer, 1988), pp. 161, 163.

56. Murphy and Elders, "Diabetes and the Black Community," pp. 123, 125–126.

57. Ibid., p. 121.

58. Ibid., pp. 121–122.

59. Ibid., p. 123; Lieberman, "Diabetes and Obesity in Elderly Black Americans," p. 152.

60. Lieberman, "Diabetes and Obesity in Elderly Black Americans," pp. 163, 166, 174; Koop, *The Surgeon General's Report on Nutrition and Health 1988,* p. 256.

61. Lieberman, "Diabetes and Obesity in Elderly Black Americans," p. 164.

62. Murphy and Elders, "Diabetes and the Black Community," pp. 122.

63. See Reed, *The Health and Medical Care of African-Americans,* p. 15; United States, *Health, United States 1993,* pp. 93–94.

64. See, Nancy R. Cope and Howard R. Hall, "Risk Factors Associated with the Health of Black Women in the United States," in Woodrow Jones and Mitchell F. Rice, eds., *Health Care Issues in Black America: Policies, Problems, and Prospects* (Westport, Conn.: Greenwood Press, 1987), pp. 43–56; Michael S. Goldstein, *The Health Movement: Promoting Fitness in America* (New York: Twayne Publishers, 1992), pp. 24–25, 141–143; Robert Staples, *The World of Black Singles: Changing Patterns of Male/Female Relations* (Westport, Conn.: Greenwood Press, 1981).

65. United States, *Health, United States 1993,* p. 82.

66. See Margaret S. Boone, *Capital Crime: Black Infant Mortality in America* (Newbury Park, Calif.: Sage, 1989), pp. 15–16, 119–120; Virginia Davis Floyd, " 'Too Soon, Too Small, Too Sick': Black Infant Mortality," in Ronald L. Braithwaite and Sandra E. Taylor, eds., *Health Issues in the Black Community* (San Francisco: Jossey-Bass, 1992), pp. 165, 167, 171–173; Koop, *The Surgeon General's Report on Nutrition and Health 1988,* p. 547.

67. United States, *Health, United States 1993,* p. 69.

68. See, for example, Floyd, " 'Too Soon, Too Small, Too Sick,' " p. 170; Wornie L. Reed, "Suffer the Children: Some Effects of Racism on the Health of Black Infants," in Peter Conrad and Rochelle Kern, eds., *The Sociology of Health and Illness: Critical Perspectives,* 2d ed. (New York: St. Martin's Press, 1986), p. 277; Ann Creighton-Zollar, *The Social Correlates of Infant and Reproductive Mortality*

in the United States: A Reference Guide (New York: Garland, 1993), pp. 36, 62, 65, 73.

69. Reed, "Suffer the Children," p. 278; Creighton-Zollar, *The Social Correlates of Infant Reproductive Mortality in the United States,* pp. 39, 93.

70. See Kiple and King, *Another Dimension to the Black Diaspora,* pp. 193–194.

71. See Creighton-Zollar, *The Social Correlates of Infant and Reproductive Mortality in the United States,* pp. 110–111, 132; Reed, "Suffer the Children," pp. 277–278.

72. Creighton-Zollar, *The Social Correlates of Infant and Reproductive Mortality in the United States,* pp. 74, 81, 100, 151.

73. Ibid., pp. 38–40, 83, 93; Reed, *The Health and Medical Care of African-Americans,* p. 21.

74. Ibid., pp. 28, 69, 73; Koop, *The Surgeon General's Report on Nutrition and Health 1988,* pp. 552–553.

75. Creigs C. Beverly, "Alcoholism and the African-American Community," in Ronald L. Braithwaite and Sandra E. Taylor, eds., *Health Issues in the Black Community* (San Francisco: Jossey-Bass, 1992), p. 79; Reed, *The Health and Medical Care of African-Americans,* p. 83; United States, Department of Health and Human Services (DHHS), Public Health Service, *Healthy People 2000: National Promotion and Disease Prevention Objectives,* DHHS Publication no. (PHS) 91–50212 (Washington D.C.: U.S. Government Printing Office, 1991), p. 164; Frederick D. Harper, "Alcohol Use and Abuse," in Lawrence E. Gary, ed., *Black Men* (Beverly Hills, Calif.: Sage, 1981), pp. 169–177.

76. Reed, *The Health and Medical Care of African Americans,* pp. 186–187; United States, *Healthy People 2000,* p. 164.

77. See Samuel V. Duh, *Blacks and Aids* (Newbury Park, Calif.: Sage, 1991); United States, *Health, United States 1993,* pp. 144, 147; Reed, *The Health and Medical Care of African-Americans,* pp. 89, 93.

78. United States, *Healthy People 2000,* p. 136; Goldstein, *The Health Movement,* p. 124.

79. Ibid.; United States, *Health, United States 1993,* p. 34; Semmes, *Cultural Hegemony and African American Development,* p. 184; United States, Environmental Protection Agency (EPA), Office of Air and Radiation, *Indoor Air Facts No. 5: Environmental Tobacco Smoke* (Washington, D.C.: U.S. EPA, Public Information Center, June 1989).

80. See E. Franklin Frazier, *Black Bourgeoisie: The Rise of a New Middle Class* (New York: Free Press, 1957), p. 171.

81. See Jannette L. Dates, "Advertising," in Jannette L. Dates and William Barlow, eds., *Split Image: African Americans in the Mass Media* (Washington, D.C.: Howard University Press, 1990), p. 436; Roberto Rodriguez, "Alcohol, Tobacco Ads: First Amendment Issue or Stranglehold on Minority Media? *Black Issues in Higher Education,* June 4, 1992, pp. 22–23; Marcus Mabry, "Fighting Ads in the Inner City," *Newsweek,* February 5, 1990, p. 115; Mark Miller, "New Tobacco Alliance," *Newsweek,* February 13, 1989, p. 113; Irwin Ross, "Push Collides with Busch," *Fortune,* November 15, 1982, pp. 90–92; Ken Smikle, "New Market for Burrell," *Black Enterprise,* January 1985, p. 29; Cornelius Foote, "Beer Facts: Stanley Scott Ices Major Miller Deal," *Black Enterprise,* June 1988, p. 41; Ira Teinowitz, "Malt Liquor Shows Muscle Despite Weak Ad Support," *Advertising*

Age, May 25, 1992, p. 12; Alan Wolf, "Malt Liquors Gain Notoriety," *Beverage World,* March 31, 1992, p. 9; Viveca Novak, "Conservatives and Corporations Plug into Black Power," *Business and Society Review,* Fall 1989, p. 32–39; Joshua Hammer and Howard Manly, "Where Black Is Gold," *Newsweek,* December 2, 1991, p. 118; Pepper Miller and Ronald Miller, "Trends Are Opportunities for Targeting African-Americans," *Marketing News,* January 20, 1992, p. 9; Beverly, "Alcoholism and the African-American Community," p. 80; Semmes, *Cultural Hegemony and African American Development,* pp. 111–138.

9

Strategies for Change: Community Action and Public Policy

There is an urgent need for a new and more effective way to view and interpret African-American health issues. To truly preserve and enhance African-American health we must shift our vision and priorities from issues related only to providing medical or sick care to constructing and institutionalizing a health ethic. This means stimulating a tradition of values and behaviors that promote and preserve the organizational basis of health in the community. I have referred to this mode of organization as the infrastructure of health; it consists of the health-related roles of family, religion, recreation, indigenous and lay health practitioners, dietary habits, environmental circumstances, and so on. Medical care is an important component of this infrastructure, but it has certain limitations and must be directed by consumers in order to serve the interest of health.

LIMITS OF MEDICINE

Many scholars, researchers, health professionals, and lay persons realize that medical care has reached certain limits in terms of reducing morbidity, mortality, and extending life. In fact, more medical care can produce, in some instances, counterproductive returns in the form of additional sickness, prohibitive costs, the atrophy of more effective determinants of health, and the dehumanization and manipulation of consumers. Those who can pay may end up with too much medical care, and those who cannot may not receive enough. The medical care that is most needed is replaced by that which is most profitable.[1]

Understanding the true basis of health, African Americans must not leave the goal of health to the market needs of a medical-industrial complex. Strengthening and empowering the family, for example, is a key objective in the struggle for African-American health and well-being. The family's role in caring, curing, prevention, establishing dietary habits, stress management, lifestyle, and the like is unparalleled. Thus, families must be aided to recognize their central importance in promoting health and taking enlightened responsibility for the therapeutic well-being of their members.

In a similar manner, we must examine the various religious traditions of which African Americans are a part to determine the extent to which these traditions may either improve or impede positive health outcomes. If religious practices lack a progressive health ethic, they should be encouraged to cultivate behaviors that enhance healthful living. Religious beliefs are powerful determinants of behavior and play a central role in the creation of new social forms. Their potential to promote better health must be tapped.

Furthermore, we must find ways to amplify the positive qualities of knowledgeable lay persons and of indigenous (folk or popular) health care practitioners who are part of the existing infrastructures of health. Regardless of the number of formally trained health professionals, there will always be those health providers who gain their legitimacy directly from the people they serve. Rather than relegate lay and indigenous health care providers to the fringe, we should recognize, respect, and seek to elevate their service to the community. Consumers and health care providers alike should have easy access to accurate and up-to-date information on which to base their health-seeking and curative decisions.

Organizing and strengthening various forms of recreation and play for children, young people, adults, and the elderly are of paramount importance. For example, a simple activity like dancing, which historically has had much importance for African-American culture, should be embraced and cultivated for its health-giving, stress-reducing, and communally cohesive properties. Historically, dance also has profound spiritual and sacred qualities, which can be developed to inspire and motivate the community to positive action. It should be advanced in appropriate and safe ways for African Americans of all ages. Culture-specific activities like jumping rope (double Dutch) and various forms of athletics can be used to promote fitness and direct youth away from at-risk behavior. The organization of healthful recreational activities for all ages must become a priority.

SELF-HELP VERSUS PUBLIC POLICY

There is an issue concerning the use of public policy versus self-help. Should government have an active role in health promotion and improving the infrastructure of health, or should a community take responsibility for its own well-being? Is the best solution to work from the bottom up or the top down? Can the private sector do a better job of promoting health than the public sector? The answer, of course, is that the public and private sector and the community must work together to achieve the goal of health. The community, however, is primary. Bottom-up relationships have the most direct affects on health. Public policy should enhance the capabilities of communities to develop and maintain viable health-giving infrastructures. A progressive community-based health ethic is critical but cannot replace necessary structural changes that need to be made in institutional, communal, and societal life. An effective health ethic is essential, however, to guide efforts to make necessary structural changes and to stimulate awareness of the need for change. Problems of economic dislocation and economic development, for example, remain basic. The pursuit of profit by the private sector should not override the goal of health.

REDUCING AND MANAGING STRESS

The characteristics of the health problems that affect the African-American community suggest that stress management and reduction efforts are extremely important. The family, of course, is the most vital support group, and the resiliency of extended family forms is especially significant to bolster the protective capabilities of fractured nuclear and single-parent families. We must also pay attention to the symbolic structures of the society and how they affect the self-image and self-esteem of African Americans. Structured inequality in the form of employment discrimination; on-the-job pressures; the daily need to negotiate unfriendly bureaucracies to obtain essential services; economic powerlessness; political dependency; the negative externalities of restricted urban living; the disproportionate exposure to environmental pollutants and hazards; poor food supplies, housing, and education; and the like lend themselves to heightened stress that affects the nutritional status and biological integrity of African Americans. Excessive stress or distress increases the rates of interpersonal conflict, violence, and homicide. The development and promotion of health arts and techniques to manage stress and conflict are necessary strategies for change.

NUTRITION AND LIFESTYLE RECOMMENDATIONS

In light of the dimensions of environmentally and status-induced stress, the character of inequality defined by cultural hegemony, and the risk factors for leading causes of morbidity and mortality among African Americans, there is a great need to define and promote specific nutritional and lifestyle recommendations for African Americans. For example, special efforts are necessary to discourage the use of added salt because of the unusually high percentage of salt-sensitive African Americans. Fresh fruit and vegetable consumption should be increased drastically to improve the sodium-potassium balance and overall nutritional density. The consumption of fat, most notably saturated fat, needs to be reduced as a proportion of total calories.

Other ethno-specific dietary recommendations and health promotion objectives are needed to address distinctive challenges to African-American health. For example, there is an obvious requirement to increase consumption of foods that are nutritionally dense in the B-complex vitamins and in vitamin C. These nutrients protect against the effects of stress. The consumption of refined sugar and empty calories from junk foods must be avoided since they destroy nutrients that protect against stress. The same is true for caffeine-laden products like coffee, colas, chocolate, and tea.

The high incidence of lactose intolerance among African Americans makes whole milk a poor source of vitamin D and calcium. Ill-suited diets also contribute to inadequate stores of vitamin D and calcium. Highly pigmented skin synthesizes vitamin D from the interaction of the sun's rays with the skin less efficiently than does skin with little pigmentation. Dark skin is protective against the sun and useful in sunny environments; less abundant sunshine presents a problem for vitamin D production. We also know that vitamin D is necessary to utilize calcium. Therefore, specific nutritional strategies should address this distinctive composite of factors. For example, promoting the consumption of fish (cod liver) oil (which is high in vitamin A and D)—especially during the winter months when the body is covered and there is less sun—as a regular part of the diet is one strategy. Providing directions for minimizing the effects of lactose intolerance (for example, consuming cultured milk products like yogurt) is another. Improving food selection and preparation to preserve nutrients, lower fat, and enhance nutritional density is also essential. Developing culturally sensitive methods to increase the availability of whole grains, whole-grain products, and fresh fruits and vegetables at low cost would be very beneficial.

In light of the deep importance of the interrelationships between stress, nutrition, maternal health, and infant mortality, a special effort must be made to alter the nutritional habits and health-related environment of potential mothers. Breast-feeding should be promoted because it provides the best nutrition for newborns and extends to infants greater immunity from disease. This effort should include altering the workplace and public spaces to provide secure and convenient locations for this healthful activity. Positive health behaviors surrounding maternal and child health must be reinforced within the family and community, and knowledge pathways from experienced and informed mothers, fathers, and elders to youth must be reopened. Age must again reflect wisdom and be a source of strength and guidance for the community.

Efforts to limit or remove alcohol, tobacco, and illicit drugs from the community must be strengthened. Moreover, community leaders and opinion makers, for example, should mount a sustained attack against the excessive ads for tobacco and alcohol that are directed at the African-American community in general and at African-American youth in particular. Schools, churches, recreational centers, barbershops and beauty parlors, libraries, block clubs, small businesses, fraternities and sororities, civic organizations, and the like should become vehicles to insulate the community against all types of drug mongers. Excessive numbers of liquor stores in African-American communities are other potential targets. Treatment for addictions and prevention programs directed at the very young should be a focus of public policy as a support for community action. Moreover, we must promote a greater awareness that even medicinal drugs should be utilized with care and only when needed. Self-reliance, self-control, and progressive health behavior can be enhanced by consumer education, social awareness, and community support.

HEALTH EDUCATION

A useful health ethic can be propagated through numerous channels in the community. One logical place is the school system. Nutritional balance, the dangers of drugs, the responsibilities of motherhood and fatherhood, human development over the life cycle, first aid and life-saving techniques, managing stress and interpersonal conflict, and avoiding sexually transmitted diseases are examples of essential health-related knowledge to which young people and others in the community should be exposed. Religious institutions can reinforce the dissemination of relevant health knowledge. Additionally, lay persons, indigenous health providers, and elders all have an important role in advancing an effective health ethic. Libraries, recreational centers, beauty parlors and barbershops, African-American bookstores, and the like are also key places to increase the visibility and awareness of important health issues and health promotion strategies. Voluntary organizations, including fraternities and sororities, should make enhancing health a key part of their collective goals and service activities. However, wherever the family can be bolstered as an effective purveyor of positive health beliefs and practices, this should be done.

Widespread efforts to bring more African Americans into the full range of health professions must increase. Young people should be exposed to careers as medical, osteopathic, and chiropractic physicians; nurses; public health professionals; dentists; optometrists; various types of therapists; nutritionists; exercise physiologists; and others at a very early age. Sustained exposure to the health professions, frequent information about how to pursue health careers, and steady encouragement to study the biological sciences should be pervasive. Ways to enrich reading, writing, math, and science skills to ensure future preparedness for training in the health professions must be a part of the goal to elevate community health. It is also the case that as the amount of education increases, so do positive health behaviors. African Americans must guard against low teacher expectations regarding the education of their children and the tendency to funnel them out of challenging curriculum tracks, particularly in integrated school settings. When there is poor preparation in a given area, the strategy should be more exposure, not less.

HEALTH ACTIVISM

Health promotion and access to low-cost and effective health care should become the new objective of Civil Rights and social activism in the African-American community. The social foundations of health are strongly influenced by patterns of inequality. Thus, the struggle to transform the health of African Americans is also the struggle to liberate this group politically, economically, and culturally. It is a battle against powerlessness and dependency. The goal of health is the kind of issue that touches all segments of the African-American community and invites the potential support of others who are interested in justice, equity, and progressive social change. A significant challenge for this social activism would be to free Civil Rights, cultural, and philanthropic organizations from their inordinate dependence on donations from tobacco and liquor companies. There is also the need to attack excessive billboard advertising by these companies in African-American communities and to reduce the pervasive presence of liquor stores.

Health activists should also work to monitor and counteract distorted and demeaning images of African Americans in the media. The media and other institutions of legitimation routinely omit the full range of accomplishments and experiences of African Americans. Blacks are cast only in certain roles, and historical accuracy that conveys the characteristics of the African-American struggle for human dignity in all phases of life is not available through normal avenues of the day-to-day constructions of reality. The effect is that African Americans lose awareness of their own resiliency, intestinal fortitude, creativity, and intelligence. Others are able to convince themselves that racial stratification does not exist, was an accident, or is a part of the natural order of things, based on the will of God or some genetic order. The psychic energy necessary to experience, respond, and transcend this perverse kind of socially constructed reality is immense and has profound consequences for African-American health. Therefore, health activism must involve sustained efforts to alter and transcend institutional arrangements that perennially contribute to the social construction and reconstruction of the myth of White supremacy.

Health activism must transform the African-American community internally, and it must transform the forces that impinge on that community's development. Such activism must involve consumer and health education; collective efforts to control guns, weapons, violence, and homicide; strategies to manage and resolve conflict; tactics to stop the sale and consumption of illicit and social drugs (alcohol and tobacco); and actions to improve maternal and child health. Activism must be directed at promoting self-help and at pressuring governmental agencies to enact policies that will improve the infrastructures of health and empower people at the institutional and community levels. Selective buying and other pressure tactics may be necessary to encourage those who market to African Americans to make sure that their products contribute to that community's health. It should become more difficult for demeaning images and destructive products to penetrate African-American communities and institutions.

Effective health activism requires the organization and support of African-American health professionals and educators. These individuals should lend their support to enlarging the health awareness, knowledge, and self-help capabilities of African-American communities through lectures, demonstrations, teaching, voluntary activity, and personal transformation. They must also be active in reforming their own professions and making them more responsive to the health needs of Black communities. These health experts must transcend professional barriers. Medical doctors, nurses, nutritionists, optometrists, chiropractors, naturopaths, herbalists, fitness instructors, Yoga teachers, lay people, and the like should be able to find a place and purpose to cooperatively advance the health of African Americans. Concentrated work with youth, mothers, children, and the elderly would be especially beneficial.

PUBLIC POLICY, FAMILY, AND MEDICAL CARE

Efforts to strengthen the family and improve other vital components of the infrastructure of health and reform medical care must proceed simultaneously. However, the trend must be for African-Americans to emphasize self-help and push for public policies that affect their specific circumstance in the context of universal determinants of health. Antipoverty efforts, job training, and business development are essential. Environmentally safe and affordable housing that encourages multigenerational families and tax incentives that encourage home and family care for the elderly are important avenues for exploration. America is faced with an increasingly aging population, and the quality of life, health, and longevity of senior citizens are enhanced when they reside in families and are involved with children. Moreover, communities must utilize more effectively the knowledge and wisdom of their senior citizens in order to stabilize and elevate family life.

Access to affordable, good-quality medical care is still not available to all Americans, and rising costs threaten to destroy the system altogether. Universal access to health care must be a goal. However, a radical alteration of the medical-industrial complex is needed. There is virtually no incentive to provide low-cost care. Rather, the trend is toward expensive, high-technology medical care, even though there is little concomitant improvement in health. Despite some evidence that managed and rationed care reduces costs initially, these cost controls are temporary.

A major problem is the lack of competition in the medical care system and the profit motive of the medical-industrial complex. Competition among medical providers is not sufficient to restrict costs. Consequently, the medical monopoly over health care must be challenged. Restrictions on the number of physicians should be eliminated. Incentives are needed to shift to the types of low-technology care that has been proven to be effective. Other health professionals, which may include chiropractors, nurse practitioners, paramedics, and midwives, should be able to provide a range of health services that previously have been reserved for medical doctors. Alternative, nonorthodox medical systems of health care should be allowed to compete and to demonstrate their ability to deliver effective, preventive, and curative health services.

Medical monopolies provide huge opportunities for corporate profits and powerful incentives for mongering. The health of the consumer remains a singular goal for many, especially for numerous dedicated health professionals, but profit is the driving force for the medical-industrial complex. Universal access to medical care may or may not become a reality; since there are few politically acceptable ways to restrict costs, the system probably will change only to preserve itself. The danger is that many people will be left without viable alternatives for sick care. Without sustained pressures for change, access to essential sick care will become increasingly restricted and maldistributed.[2]

Some options for African Americans are to demand a more competitive and open marketplace, become more educated and aware consumers, stress preventive measures and self-help, and seek universal access to sick care for all people, while pushing for radical restructuring of the medical system to limit costs and promote health. There are also special needs, which include emergency and prenatal care. For example, the current social conditions necessitate significant resources to address emergencies related to drug abuse, accidents, and violence-related injuries. Low-cost prenatal care should be available because of its proven effectiveness in mitigating low-birth-weight pregnancies, a major risk factor in infant mortality.

One way to limit costs is to direct the medical system to utilize minimal amounts of diagnostic technology and to develop stringent guidelines for utilizing drug therapy and surgery. Consumer, community, and Civil Rights groups, however, also must act to monitor unnecessary medical interventions and encourage individuals and families to become more involved in the caring and curing processes. Regardless of how the medical system responds to the crisis of cost, African Americans must proactively respond to their distinctive health care needs and develop strategies to enhance the infrastructures of health that govern their well-being.

CRITICAL SOURCES OF A MODEL FOR ACTION

The foundations of a model for advancing the goal of health in the African-American community already exist. The National Negro Health Week movement, initiated by Booker T. Washington in 1915, forms one part of this model. This endeavor should be revived as the National African-American Health Movement. Traditionally celebrated during the eight-day period (Sunday to Sunday) that included April 5 (Booker T. Washington's birthday), Negro Health Week galvanized African-American communities to promote health education, health awareness, and self-help, health activities and should be expanded to include the entire month of April. Through organizations representing all phases of African-American life, Washington's health movement attempted to reach all African Americans to teach them how to improve their health conditions and to lessen deaths and sickness. The specific objectives were:

(1) To provide practical suggestions for the local Health Week Committees that conduct the observance, and (2) to stimulate the people as a whole to cooperative endeavor in clean-up, educational, and specific hygienic and clinical services for general sanitary improvement of the community and for health betterment of the individual, family, and home.[3]

National Negro Health News was an extraordinary publication, first published at Tuskegee, and then by the United States Public Health Service in 1921. It provided viable objectives and strategies to carry out health reforms in African-American communities. The publication became the vehicle to guide local Health Week Committees in the observance of Health Week. Community leaders awarded medals and trophies to stimulate local activities and the participation of school children (for example, a Health Week poster contest became customary). *National Negro Health News* also published annual statistics on the activities and accomplishments of Health Week.[4] It carried an exceptional array of articles advancing strategies for improving the health of the African-American community. For example, one article offered a strategy for improving the health of

African-Americans by integrating nutritional education with the curriculum of young school children.[5]

The renewal of a national African-American health initiative would require significant modification from the earlier effort. African-American studies departments, centers, and programs, perhaps, could take the lead in such an endeavor. African-American health professionals are another possibility. A national, community-based health initiative, however, should not be dominated by the medical and pharmaceutical establishment but should enhance broad cooperation among all groups and individuals who can effect meaningful change. At the very least, the National Negro Health Week model and its principle organ, *National Negro Health News,* should be scrutinized for its progressive elements. Any new endeavors similarly must stimulate broad community awareness and involvement and must enlarge the capacity for self-help.

A second component of a model for action must come from the lessons of the alternative health movement associated with the Black Consciousness movement of the late 1960s and 1970s. First, this movement correctly connected health with self-help, self-improvement, self-determination, and enlightened cultural change. Second, it served to revitalize traditional African values (but in new configurations) that advocated a more holistic view (involving the integration of mind, body, and spirit) of health that revealed the importance of environmental, interpersonal, and spiritual balance. This health awareness and reconnection to an integrated and more satisfying identity had a galvanizing effect that moved many African Americans to make positive health-related changes. These efforts were not without their problems, but they spawned an important and essential search for a better way of life. Third, the movement provided a necessary critique of medical-industrial practices, which tend to advance the goal of profit rather than the goal of health. Indeed the tendency of the alternative health movement to advance a psychosocial-spiritual model of health incorporates the more effective view that health is a function of diverse psychological, social, and cultural processes that affect the integrity of the human body. The metaproblem of cultural hegemony, which perennially destabilizes progressive institutional and cultural development among African Americans, and the added disruptive aspects of a post-industrial order require, with some urgency, the implementation of a comprehensive, community-based health ethic.

NOTES

1. See for example, Robert G. Evans and G. L. Stoddart, "Producing Health, Consuming Health Care," in Robert G. Evans, Morris L. Baer, and Theodore R. Marmor, eds., *Why Are Some People Healthy and Others Not? The Determinants of Health of Populations* (New York: Aldine DeGruyter, 1994), pp. 27–64; Michael

S. Goldstein, *The Health Movement: Promoting Fitness in America* (New York: Twayne Publishers, 1992), pp. 2–11.

2. See the collection of articles in Martin A. Strosberg, Joshua M. Wiener, Robert Baker, and I. Alan Fein, eds., *Rationing America's Medical Care: The Oregon Plan and Beyond* (Washington, D.C.: Brookings Institution, 1992).

3. Roscoe C. Brown, "The National Negro Health Week Movement," *Journal of Negro Education* 6 (July 1937): 555.

4. See the July–September issues of this quarterly publication.

5. See Olive Welbourne and Dorothy Bovee, "Readin', Ritin', Rithmetic, and Right Eatin'," *National Negro Health News* 18 (January–March 1950): 5–8.

Selected Bibliography

Afrika, Llaila O. *African Holistic Health.* 3d ed. Silver Spring, Md.: Sea Island Information Group, 1983.

Andritzky, Walter, ed. *Yearbook of Cross-Cultural Medicine and Psychotherapy 1992.* Berlin, Germany: International Institute of Cross-Cultural Therapy Research, 1994.

Angel, Ronald, and Jacqueline Lowe Worobey. "Single Motherhood and Children's Health." *Journal of Health and Social Behavior* 29 (March 1988): 38–52.

Asante, Molefi Kete. *Kemet, Afrocentricity and Knowledge.* Trenton, N.J.: Africa World Press, 1990.

Bachrach, Steven, Julian Fisher, and John S. Parks. "An Outbreak of Vitamin D Deficiency Rickets in a Susceptible Population." *Pediatrics* 64, no. 6 (December 1979): 871–877.

Baer, Hans A. "Prophets and Advisors in Black Spiritual Churches: Therapy, Palliative, or Opiate?" *Culture, Medicine and Psychiatry* 5 (1981): 145–170.

———. "Toward a Systematic Typology of Black Folk Healers." *Phylon* 43 (1982): 327–343.

Bailey, Eric J. *Urban African American Health Care.* Lanham, Md.: University Press of America, 1991.

Bastide, Roger. "Color, Racism, and Christianity." In *Color and Race,* ed. John Hope Franklin. Boston: Beacon Press, 1969, pp. 34–49.

Beckles, Hilary, and Verene Shepherd, eds. *Caribbean Slave Society and Economy.* New York: New Press, 1991.

Bennett, Lerone, Jr. *Confrontation: Black and White.* Baltimore, Md.: Penguin Books, 1966.

Berg, Alan. *The Nutrition Factor: Its Role in National Development.* Washington, D.C.: Brookings Institution, 1973.

Berkley, George. *On Being Black and Healthy: How Black Americans Can Lead Longer and Healthier Lives.* Englewood Cliffs, N.J.: Prentice-Hall, 1982.

Billingsley, Andrew. *Climbing Jacob's Ladder: The Enduring Legacy of African-American Families.* New York: Simon and Schuster, 1992.

Blake, J. Herman. " 'Doctor Can't Do Me No Good': Social Concomitants of Health Care Attitudes and Practices among Elderly Blacks in Isolated Rural Populations." In *Black Folk Medicine: The Therapeutic Significance of Faith and Trust,* ed. Wilbur H. Watson. New Brunswick, N.J.: Transaction Books, 1984, pp. 33–40.

Blassingame, John W. *The Slave Community.* Rev. ed. New York: Oxford University Press, 1979.

Boone, Margaret S. *Capital Crime: Black Infant Mortality in America.* Newbury Park, Calif.: Sage, 1989.

Boyd, Eddie L., Leslie A. Shimp, and Marvie Jarmon Hackney. *Home Remedies and the Black Elderly: A Reference Manual for Health Care Providers.* Ann Arbor: University of Michigan, Institute of Gerontology and College of Pharmacy, 1984.

Braithwaite, Ronald L., and Sandra E. Taylor, eds. *Health Issues in the Black Community.* San Francisco: Jossey-Bass, 1992.

Brown, Roscoe C. "The National Negro Health Week Movement." *Journal of Negro Education* 6 (July 1937): 553–564.

Bryant, Bunyan, and Paul Mohai, eds. *Race and the Incidence of Environmental Hazards: A Time for Discourse.* Boulder, Colo.: Westview Press, 1992.

Butler, John Sibley. *Entrepreneurship and Self-Help among Black Americans: A Reconsideration of Race and Economics.* New York: State University of New York Press, 1991.

Carew, Jan. "Columbus and the Origins of Racism in the Americas: Part One." *Race and Class* 29 (Spring 1988): 1–19.

———. "Columbus and the Origins of Racism in the Americas: Part Two." *Race and Class* 30 (July–September 1988): 33–57.

Carruthers, Jacob H. *MAAT: The African Universe.* Chicago: Center for Inner City Studies, 1979.

Carter, Shirley A. Vaughn. "Reflections on Equal Educational Opportunity in Baccalaureate Nursing Programs." *Western Journal of Black Studies* 9 (Fall 1985): 152–157.

Chivian, Eric, Michael McCally, Howard Hu, and Andrew Haines, eds. *Critical Condition: Human Health and the Environment: A Report by Physicians for Social Responsibility.* Cambridge, Mass.: Massachusetts Institute of Technology Press, 1993.

Conniff, Michael L., and Thomas J. Davis. *Africans in the Americas: A History of the Black Diaspora.* New York: St. Martin's Press, 1994.

Conrad, Peter, and Rochelle Kern, eds. *The Sociology of Health and Illness: Critical Perspectives.* 2d ed. New York: St. Martin's Press, 1986.

Cotton, Dorothy H. G. *Stress Management: An Integrated Approach to Therapy.* New York: Brunner/Mazel, 1990.

Creighton-Zollar, Ann. *The Social Correlates of Infant and Reproductive Mortality in the United States: A Reference Guide.* New York: Garland, 1993.

Curtin, Philip, ed. *Africa Remembered: Narratives by West Africans from the Era of the Slave Trade.* Madison: University of Wisconsin Press, 1967.

Dates, Jannette L., and William Barlow, eds. *Split Image: African Americans in the Mass Media.* Washington, D.C.: Howard University Press, 1990.

Davidson, Basil. *The African Slave Trade: Precolonial History 1450–1850.* Boston: Little, Brown and Company, 1961.

———. *Modern Africa: A Social and Political History.* 2d ed. New York: Longman, 1989.

deGraft-Johnson, J. C. *African Glory: The Story of Vanished Negro Civilizations.* Baltimore, Md.: Black Classic Press, 1986.

Diop, Cheikh Anta. *The African Origin of Civilization: Myth or Reality.* Westport, Conn.: Lawrence Hill, 1974.

———. *Civilization or Barbarism: An Authentic Anthropology.* Brooklyn, N.Y.: Lawrence Hill, 1991.

Doherty, William J., and Thomas L. Campbell. *Families and Health.* Beverly Hills, Calif.: Sage, 1988.

Doyle, Bertram. *The Etiquette of Race Relations in the South: A Study in Social Control.* New York: Schocken Books, 1971.

Drake, St. Clair. *Black Folk Here and There: An Essay in History and Anthropology.* Vol. 2. Los Angeles: University of California, Center for Afro-American Studies, 1990.

Drake, St. Clair, and Horace R. Cayton. *Black Metropolis: A Study of Negro Life in a Northern City.* Vol. 1. Rev. ed. New York: Harper and Row, 1962.

Du Bois, W.E.B. *Dusk of Dawn: An Essay toward an Autobiography of a Race Concept.* New York: Schocken Books, 1968.

———. *The Negro American Family.* Atlanta University Publications, no. 13. Atlanta, Ga.: Atlanta University Press, 1908.

———. *The Philadelphia Negro: A Social Study.* New York: Schocken Books, 1967.

———. *The Souls of Black Folk.* Greenwich, Conn.: Fawcett, 1961.

Duffy, John. *The Healers: A History of American Medicine.* Chicago: University of Illinois Press, 1979.

Duh, Samuel V. *Blacks and Aids.* Newbury Park, Calif.: Sage, 1991.

Ehrenreich, Barbara, and Deirdre English. *Witches, Midwives, and Nurses: A History of Women Healers.* New York: Feminist Press, 1973.

Ellis, John. *The Social History of the Machine Gun.* New York: Pantheon, 1975.

Evans, Robert G., Morris L. Baer, and Theodore R. Marmor, eds. *Why Are Some People Healthy and Others Not? The Determinants of Health of Populations.* New York: Aldine DeGruyter, 1994.

Fanon, Franz. *Black Skin, White Mask.* New York: Grove Press, 1967.

Farley, Reynolds, and Walter R. Allen. *The Color Line and the Quality of Life in America.* New York: Oxford University Press, 1989.

Franklin, John Hope, and Alfred A. Moss, Jr. *From Slavery to Freedom: A History of Negro Americans.* 6th ed. New York: McGraw-Hill, 1988.

Frazier, E. Franklin. *Black Bourgeoisie: The Rise of a New Middle Class.* New York: Free Press, 1957.

———. *The Negro Church in America.* New York: Schocken Books, 1966.

———. *The Negro Family in the United States.* Rev. ed. Chicago: University of Chicago Press, 1966.

———. *Race and Culture Contacts in the Modern World.* Boston: Beacon Press, 1957.

Frohock, Fred M. *Healing Powers: Alternative Medicine, Spiritual Communities and the State.* Chicago: University of Chicago Press, 1992.

Fuchs, Victor R. *The Health Economy.* Cambridge, Mass.: Harvard University Press, 1986.

Genovese, Eugene. *Roll Jordan Roll: The World the Slaves Made.* New York: Vintage Books, 1976.

George, Susan. *How the Other Half Dies: The Real Reasons for World Hunger.* Montclair, N.J.: Allanfeld, Osmun and Company, 1977.

Ginzburg, Ralph. *100 Years of Lynchings.* Baltimore, Md.: Black Classic Press, 1988.

Goldstein, Michael S. *The Health Movement: Promoting Fitness in America.* New York: Twayne Publishers, 1992.

González-Wippler, Migene. *Santeria: African Magic in Latin America.* New York: Original Publications, 1987.

Goodson, Martia Graham. "Medical-Botanical Contributions of African Slave Women to American Medicine." *Western Journal of Black Studies* 11 (Winter 1987): 198–203.

Gregory, Dick. *Dick Gregory's Natural Diet for Folks Who Eat: Cookin' with Mother Nature.* New York: Harper and Row, 1973.

Harper, Frederick D. "Alcohol Use and Abuse." In *Black Men,* ed. Lawrence E. Gary. Beverly Hills, Calif.: Sage, 1981, pp. 169–177.

Hartwig, Gerald W., and K. David Patterson, eds. *Disease in African History: An Introductory Survey and Case Studies.* Durham, N.C.: Duke University Press, 1978.

Hawkins, Darnell F., ed. *Homicide among Black Americans.* Lanham, Md.: University Press of America, 1986.

Henri, Florette. *Black Migration: Movement North 1900–1920.* Garden City, N.Y.: Anchor Press/Doubleday, 1975.

Hernton, Calvin C. *Sex and Racism in America.* New York: Grove Press, 1966.

Hilliard, Sam Bowers. *Hog Meat and Hoecake: Food Supply in the Old South, 1840–1860.* Carbondale: Southern Illinois University Press, 1972.

Hine, Darlene Clark. *Black Women in White: Racial Conflict and Cooperation in the Nursing Profession 1890–1950.* Bloomington: Indiana University Press, 1989.

Holloway, Joseph E., ed. *Africanisms in American Culture.* Bloomington: Indiana University Press, 1990.

Horton, Robin. "African Traditional Thought and Western Science." *Africa* 37 (1967): 50–71.

Hurston, Zora. "Hoodoo in America." *Journal of American Folk-Lore* 44 (October–December 1931): 317–417.

Illich, Ivan. *Medical Nemesis: The Expropriation of Health.* New York: Pantheon, 1976.

Iyi, Kilindi. "African Roots in Asian Martial Arts." In *African Presence in Early*

Asia, ed. Ivan Van Sertima and Runoko Rashidi. New Brunswick, N.J.: Transaction Books, 1988, pp. 138–143.

Jackson, Bruce. "The Other Kind of Doctor: Conjure and Magic in Black American Folk Medicine." In *American Folk Medicine: A Symposium,* ed. Wayland D. Hand. Los Angeles: University of California Press, 1976, pp. 259–272.

Jackson, James S., ed. *The Black American Elderly: Research on Physical and Psychosocial Health.* New York: Springer, 1988.

Jackson, John G. *Man, God, and Civilization.* New Hyde Park, N.Y.: University Books, 1972.

Johnson, Charles S. *Shadow of the Plantation.* Chicago: University of Chicago Press, 1966.

Johnson, Daniel M., and Rex R. Campbell. *Black Migration in America: A Social Demographic History.* Durham, N.C.: Duke University Press, 1981.

Johnson, James H., Jr., and Melvin L. Oliver. "Blacks and the Toxic Crisis." *Western Journal of Black Studies* 13, no. 2 (Summer 1989): 72–78.

Jones, Jacqueline. *Labor of Love, Labor of Sorrow: Black Women, Work and the Family, From Slavery to the Present.* New York: Vintage Books, 1986.

Jones, James H. *Bad Blood: The Tuskegee Syphilis Experiment—A Tragedy of Race and Medicine.* New York: Free Press, 1981.

Jones, Norrece T., Jr. *Born a Child of Freedom, Yet a Slave: Mechanisms of Control and Strategies of Resistance in Antebellum South Carolina.* Hanover, N.H. and London: University Press of New England, 1990.

Jones, Woodrow, and Mitchell F. Rice, eds. *Health Care Issues in Black America: Policies, Problems, and Prospects.* Westport, Conn.: Greenwood Press, 1987.

Jordan, Winthrop. *White over Black: American Attitudes toward the Negro 1550–1812.* Baltimore, Md.: Penguin Books, 1969.

Kane, Robert L., ed. *The Challenge of Community Medicine.* New York: Springer, 1974.

Kiple, Kenneth F. *The Caribbean Slave: A Biological History.* New York: Cambridge University Press, 1984.

Kiple, Kenneth F., ed. *The African Exchange: Toward a Biological History of Black People.* Durham, N.C.: Duke University Press, 1987.

Kiple, Kenneth F., and Virginia Himmelsteib King. *Another Dimension to the Black Diaspora: Diet, Disease, and Racism.* New York: Cambridge University Press, 1981.

Koop, C. Everett. *The Surgeon General's Report on Nutrition and Health 1988.* Rocklin, Calif.: Prima Publishing and Communications, 1989.

Kosa, John, and Irving Kenneth Zola, eds. *Poverty and Health: A Sociological Analysis.* Cambridge, Mass.: Harvard University Press, 1975.

Kowalchik, Claire, and William H. Hylton, eds. *Rodale's Illustrated Encyclopedia of Herbs.* Emmaus, Pa.: Rodale Press, 1987.

Lambo, J. O. "The Impact of Colonialism on African Cultural Heritage with Special Reference to the Practice of Herbalism in Nigeria." In *Traditional Healing,* ed. Philip Singer. New York: Conch Magazine Limited, 1977, pp. 123–135.

Landry, Bart. *The New Black Middle Class.* Berkeley and Los Angeles: University of California Press, 1987.

Lee, Anne S., and Everett S. Lee. "The Health of Slaves and the Health of Freedmen: A Savannah Study." *Phylon* 38 (1977): 170–178.

Lewicki, Tadeuz. *West African Food in the Middle Ages: According to Arabic Sources.* New York: Cambridge University Press, 1974.

Lewis, David Levering. *W.E.B. Du Bois: Biography of a Race 1868–1919.* New York: Henry Holt, 1993.

Lewis, Hylan. *Blackways of Kent.* New Haven, Conn.: College and University Press, 1964.

Livingston, Ivor Lensworth, ed. *Handbook of Black American Health: The Mosaic of Conditions, Issues, Policies, and Prospects.* Westport, Conn.: Greenwood Press, 1994.

Luckert, Karl W. *Egyptian Light and Hebrew Fire: Theological and Philosophical Roots of Christendom in Evolutionary Perspective.* Albany: State University of New York Press, 1991.

Martin, Elmer P., and Joanne Mitchell Martin. *The Black Extended Family.* Chicago: University of Chicago Press, 1978.

Maynard, Aubre L. *Surgeon to the Poor: The Harlem Hospital Story.* New York: Appleton-Century-Crofts, 1978.

Mbiti, John S. *African Religions and Philosophy.* 2d ed. Oxford: Heinemann, 1990.

McBride, David. *From TB to AIDS: Epidemics among Urban Blacks since 1900.* Albany: State University of New York Press, 1991.

McGuire, Meredith B. *Ritual Healing in Suburban America.* New Brunswick, N.J.: Rutgers University Press, 1988.

Mendelsohn, Robert S. *Male Practice: How Doctors Manipulate Women.* Chicago: Contemporary Books, 1982.

Mokhtar, Gamal el Din, ed. *The UNESCO General History of Africa II: Ancient Civilizations of Africa.* Abr. ed. Berkeley: University of California Press, 1990.

Moore, Barrington, Jr. *Social Origins of Dictatorship and Democracy: Lord and Peasant in the Making of the Modern World.* Boston: Beacon Press, 1966.

Morais, Herbert M. *The History of the Negro in Medicine.* New York: Publishers Company, 1967.

Morse, Donald R., and Robert L. Pollack. *Nutrition, Stress, and Aging: A Holistic Approach to the Relationship among Stress and Food Selection, Digestion, Nutrients, Body Weight, Disease, and Longevity.* New York: AMS Press, 1988.

Mphande, Lupenga, and Linda James-Myers. "Traditional African Medicine and the Optimal Theory: Universal Insights for Health and Healing." *Journal of Black Psychology* 19 (February 1993): 25–47.

National Research Council Committee on the Status of Black Americans. *A Common Destiny: Blacks and American Society.* Washington, D.C.: National Academy Press, 1989.

Newsome, Frederick. "Black Contributions to the Early History of Western Medicine." *Journal of African Civilizations* 2 (September 1980): 27–39.

Niane, D. T. *General History of Africa. Vol. 4, Africa from the Twelfth to the Sixteenth Century.* Paris and London: United Nations Educational, Scientific, and Cultural Organization and Heineman Educational Books, 1984.

Odejide, A. O., M. O. Olatawura, A. O. Sanda, and A. O. Oyeneye. "Traditional

Healers and Mental Illness in the City of Ibadan." *Journal of Black Studies* 9 (December 1978): 195–205.

Olela, Henry. *From Ancient Africa to Ancient Greece: An Introduction to the History of Philosophy.* Atlanta, Ga.: Black Heritage Corporation, 1981.

Osofsky, Gilbert. *Harlem: The Making of a Ghetto, Negro New York, 1890–1930.* New York: Harper and Row, 1966.

Payer, Lynn. *Disease-Mongers: How Doctors, Drug Companies, and Insurers Are Making You Feel Sick.* New York: John Wiley and Son, 1992.

Payne-Jackson, Arvilla, and John Lee. *Folk Wisdom and Mother Wit: John Lee— An African American Herbal Healer.* Westport, Conn.: Greenwood Press, 1993.

Piersen, William D. *Black Legacy: America's Hidden Heritage.* Amherst: University of Massachusetts Press, 1993.

Postell, William Dosite. *The Health of Slaves on Southern Plantations.* Gloucester, Mass.: Peter Smith, 1970.

Powdermaker, Hortense. *After Freedom: A Cultural Study in the Deep South.* New York: Russell and Russell, 1968.

Puckett, Newbell Niles. *Folk Beliefs of the Southern Negro.* Chapel Hill: University of North Carolina Press, 1926.

Raboteau, Albert J. *Slave Religion: The "Invisible Institution" in the Antebellum South.* Oxford, U.K.: Oxford University Press, 1980.

Raper, Arthur R. *Preface to Peasantry: A Tale of Two Black Belt Counties.* New York: Antheneum, 1968.

———. *The Tragedy of Lynching.* New York: Dover Publications, 1970.

Reed, Wornie L. *The Health and Medical Care of African-Americans.* Boston: University of Massachusetts at Boston, William Monroe Trotter Institute, 1992.

Relman, Arnold S. "The New Medical-Industrial Complex." *New England Journal of Medicine* 303 (October 23, 1980): 963–970.

Rodney, Walter. *How Europe Underdeveloped Africa.* Dar es Salaam, Tanzania: Tanzania Publishing House, 1972.

Rose, Harold M., and Paula D. McClain. *Race, Place, and Risk: Black Homicide in Urban America.* Albany: State University of New York Press, 1990.

Rose, Margaret A. *The Post-Modern and the Post-Industrial: A Critical Analysis.* New York: Cambridge University Press, 1991.

Savitt, Todd L. *Medicine and Slavery: The Diseases and Health Care of Blacks in Antebellum Virginia.* Chicago: University of Illinois Press, 1978.

Scully, Diana. *Men Who Control Women's Health: The Miseducation of Obstetrician Gynecologists.* Boston: Houghton Mifflin, 1980.

Seham, Max. *Blacks and American Medical Care.* Minneapolis: University of Minnesota Press, 1973.

Semmes, Clovis E. *Cultural Hegemony and African American Development.* Westport, Conn.: Praeger, 1992.

Sheridan, Richard B. *Doctors and Slaves: A Medical and Demographic History of Slavery in the British West Indies, 1680–1834.* Cambridge: Cambridge University Press, 1985.

Sloan, Patricia. "Early Black Nursing Schools and Responses of Black Nurses to

Their Educational Programs." *Western Journal of Black Studies* 9 (Fall 1985): 158–172.

Smith, Jonathan C. *Understanding Stress and Coping.* New York: Macmillan, 1993.

Snow, Loudell F. *Walkin' over Medicine.* Boulder, Colo.: Westview Press, 1993.

Sobel, David, ed. *Ways of Health: Holistic Approaches to Ancient and Contemporary Medicine.* New York: Harcourt, Brace, Jovanovich, 1979.

Spear, Allan H. *Black Chicago: The Making of a Negro Ghetto, 1890–1920.* Chicago: University of Chicago Press, 1967.

Spicer, Edward H., ed. *Ethnic Medicine in the Southwest.* Tucson: University of Arizona Press, 1977.

Stampp, Kenneth M. *The Peculiar Institution: Slavery in the Ante-Bellum South.* New York: Vintage Books, 1956.

Stanfield, John H. "Venereal Disease Control Demonstrations among Rural Blacks in the American South." *Western Journal of Black Studies* 5 (Winter 1981): 246–253.

Staples, Robert. *The World of Black Singles: Changing Patterns of Male/Female Relations.* Westport, Conn.: Greenwood Press, 1981.

Starr, Paul. *The Social Transformation of American Medicine: The Rise of a Sovereign Profession and the Making of a Vast Industry.* New York: Basic Books, 1982.

Stuckey, Sterling. *Going through the Storm: The Influence of African American Art in History.* New York: Oxford University Press, 1994.

———. *Slave Culture: Nationalist Theory and the Foundations of Black America.* Oxford, U.K.: Oxford University Press, 1987.

Thompson, Vincent Bakpetu. *The Making of the African Diaspora in the Americans 1441–1900.* New York: Longman, 1987.

U.S. Bureau of the Census. *The Social and Economic Status of the Black Population in the United States: An Historical View, 1790–1978.* Current Population Reports, Special Studies Series P-23, no. 80. Washington, D.C.: U.S. Government Printing Office, 1979.

Waitzkin, Howard. *The Second Sickness: Contradictions of Capitalist Health Care.* New York: Free Press, 1983.

Watson, Wilbur H., ed. *Black Folk Medicine: The Therapeutic Significance of Faith and Trust.* New Brunswick, N.J.: Transaction Books, 1984.

Welsing, Frances Cress. *The Isis Papers: The Keys to the Colors.* Chicago: Third World Press, 1991.

Wilkinson, Doris Y., and Marvin B. Sussman, eds. *Alternative Health Maintenance and Healing Systems for Families.* New York: Haworth Press, 1987.

Williams, Richard Allen, ed. *Textbook of Black-Related Diseases.* New York: McGraw-Hill, 1975.

Willis, David P., ed. *Health Policies and Black Americans.* New Brunswick, N.J.: Transaction Publishers, 1989.

Woodson, Carter G. *A Century of Negro Migration.* New York: Russell and Russell, 1969.

Index

About the Author

CLOVIS E. SEMMES (aka Jabulani Kamau Makalani) is Professor of African American Studies at Eastern Michigan University. His teaching and research focus on African-American institutions and culture, inequality, and health and illness behavior. Dr. Semmes is known for his elaborative work in cultural hegemony as a metaproblem shaping the field of African-American studies. He has published numerous scholarly articles and is author of the book *Cultural Hegemony and African American Development* (Praeger, 1992).